The Core Concepts of OCCUPATIONAL THERAPY

of related interest

Creative Coping Skills for Children
Emotional Support through Arts and Crafts Activities
Bonnie Thomas
ISBN 978 1 84310 921 1

Exploring the Self through Photography
Activities for Use in Group Work
Claire Craig
ISBN 978 1 84310 666 1

Yoga for Children with Autism Spectrum Disorders
A Step-by-Step Guide for Parents and Caregivers
Dion E. Betts and Stacey W. Betts
ISBN 978 1 84310 817 7

Activities for Adults with Learning Disabilities
Having Fun, Meeting Needs
Helen Sonnet and Ann Taylor
ISBN 978 1 84310 975 4

The Core Concepts of OCCUPATIONAL THERAPY

A Dynamic Framework for Practice

Jennifer Creek
Foreword by Anne Lawson-Porter

Jessica Kingsley Publishers
London and Philadelphia

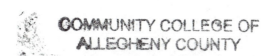

First published in 2010
by Jessica Kingsley Publishers
116 Pentonville Road
London N1 9JB, UK
and
400 Market Street, Suite 400
Philadelphia, PA 19106, USA

www.jkp.com

Library of Congress Cataloging in Publication Data
A CIP catalog record for this book is available from the Library of Congress

British Library Cataloguing in Publication Data
A CIP catalogue record for this book is available from the British Library

ISBN 978 1 84905 007 4

Printed and bound in Great Britain by
MPG Books Limited

ACKNOWLEDGEMENTS

This book has been published with the support of grant 223102-CP-1-2005-1-NL-ERASMUS-TN from the European Commission through the Socrates/Erasmus programme for Thematic Networks.

The publication is based on work undertaken as part of the terminology project, which was supported by the European Network of Occupational Therapy in Higher Education (ENOTHE) over the period 2005–2008.

The author would like to acknowledge the contributions of her fellow members of the ENOTHE terminology project working group to preparing the book outline: Miguel Brea, Joaquim Faias, Hilde Pitteljon, Sylvie Meyer and Johanna Stadler-Grillmaier. Without their expertise and dedication, the book could not have been written. The author would also like to thank three people who generously gave their time to read and comment on drafts of the text: Juanita Payne, Anne Lawson-Porter and Suzanne Wood.

Finally, the author would like to thank Hanneke van Bruggen for inviting her to participate in the ENOTHE terminology project.

CONTENTS

FOREWORD

I am delighted to have been asked to write the foreword for this European occupational therapy terminology book. I feel I have a connection with it, having been a member of various ENOTHE workshops that have explored the concepts herein. I recall at one particular workshop having my brain 'stretched' when being asked to consider such things as 'When is something that you do a task, an activity, an occupation or a chore? What are the circumstances, perceptions and perspectives that influence how you view what you are doing?' These are very complex questions that require considerable thought in any language, let alone across the breadth of languages in Europe where some words do not exist at all and others have political or sensitive connotations.

I am reminded of an author, Estelle Breines, who published an article in the *British Journal of Occupational Therapy* entitled 'Understanding occupation as the founders did'. It became one of those key works for me that situated my understanding of the concept of occupation as a mind/body phenomenon with spatial, temporal and social perspectives. This European publication, by comparison, has moved my understanding forward by miles.

The terminology group that has worked to produce this book has taken eight years to do so. In that time there has been considerable research of literature and a systematic approach to understanding terms and their use in everyday and occupational therapy language before then reaching a consensus definition. The group's work, however, did not stop there as the group realized that consensus definitions, whilst helpful, do not give an appreciation of the whole picture. The group went on to explore the relationships between the terms and the factors that influence how the terms are enacted by individuals and groups. The result is a well written, methodical exposition of professional language, illustrated by some astutely observed examples of how people demonstrate and explain these concepts in their every day lives. For me, these examples bring this book to life and have helped me to see and understand the complex inter-relationships between what people do, how they do it, why they do it and the limiting factors that sometimes impinge on their desired outcomes.

This book does what it says: 'it is a structure for the organization of professional knowledge, not a framework, not hierarchical – a dynamic, complex structure that can accommodate the flexibility of expert occupational therapy practice'. It is both fascinating and challenging and needs to be approached with thoughtfulness and reflection. It will provide a vehicle through which occupational therapists will more clearly be able to explain their interventions with people and the dynamic and complex factors that affect those interventions. I feel it will become a seminal piece of work and I therefore would wish to see this book on every undergraduate reading list and on every department's bookshelf as a reference for analysing and reflecting on the interplay between environment, personal factors, what is being done and the impact on the individual.

We all read extensively in our professional lives. You will all be able to recall those articles and books that have been the most influential in developing your thinking. You may also recognize that those influential texts can most probably be counted on the digits of two hands. This book will be one of my ten most influential texts and I commend the working group for adding to occupational therapy's body of knowledge.

Anne Lawson-Porter
Head of Education and Learning,
College of Occupational Therapists,
London,
July 2009

PREFACE

I have been an occupational therapist for nearly 40 years and have, for most of that time, been fascinated by the difficulties that occupational therapists appear to have with their professional language. The first conference paper I presented, in 1992, was called 'Why can't occupational therapists say what they do?'

In 2003, I was introduced to Hanneke van Bruggen at a national conference, in Glasgow. Until that point, I had not heard of the European Network of Occupational Therapy in Higher Education (ENOTHE). Hanneke knew of my interest in professional language and invited me to join the ENOTHE terminology working group. She said that this would involve an expenses-paid trip to Prague to meet the other group members, and subsequent meetings in other European cities. Despite not really believing that this was a genuine offer, I agreed to join the group. A few months later, I found myself in Prague, meeting four of the other group members.

When I joined the terminology working group, they had already designed a method for selecting and defining key terms, and had produced the first consensus definitions. Everyone in the group spoke fluent English and they made me very welcome. Our first meeting was a revelation – here was a group of people who, like me, could happily spend an entire afternoon discussing the finer points of meaning of a single word! These were occupational therapists who shared my own passion for language and communication.

The first terminology project lasted for three years but all of us wanted to continue with the work. We submitted a second project proposal, based on our realization that the terms we were defining represented all the concepts that underpin occupational therapy theory and practice. The new project was to construct a conceptual framework that would show how occupational therapy concepts relate to each other and how they can be used to explain the dynamic, complex nature of occupational therapy intervention.

As a multinational, multilingual group, we were strongly aware of the importance of using culturally appropriate language in occupational therapy. We felt that our profession suffers from the dominance of North American theory, which has often been adopted by occupational therapists in other English-speaking countries without thorough critical appraisal, and has been translated into other languages in a similarly uncritical way. We thought that the European conceptual framework should not be written in English and subsequently translated into the other languages of the group, but should be written from scratch in each of those languages.

To this end, we decided that each of us would write a book about the framework, in our own language and using our own culturally appropriate references. We would take responsibility for finding publishers in our own countries and, if possible, the six versions of the book would be published simultaneously. We were very ambitious!

During the second terminology project, the group met twice or three times a year, sometimes at ENOTHE events but also independently. We found that Belgium was a convenient place for us to reach and held several meetings there, finding the home of our Belgian colleague a welcoming place in which to continue our ongoing dialogue. At these meetings, we wrote detailed outlines of the book chapters, so that all six versions of the book would be written to the same template. Back at home, we started writing the book, discussing the progress and challenges when we met again.

ENOTHE conferences provided a forum for sharing the work in progress with occupational therapy teachers from many European countries, through a series of workshops. The critical discussions that took place at these events shaped the way that we wrote the book, as people told us how best to communicate the dynamic nature of the conceptual framework. We were heartened to find that the many occupational therapy lecturers who attended these workshops not only understood the framework but were extremely enthusiastic about it.

For me, the European conceptual framework for occupational therapy represents the culmination of almost 40 years of thinking, talking and writing about the language of occupational therapy. The framework does not attempt to simplify the complexity of human doing by using words that lock activities and occupations into static categories. Rather, it captures the dynamism and unpredictability of occupation in all its manifestations.

This book is one of six versions, written in six languages, that explain the professional terminology of occupational therapy for European theory and practice. It is the outcome of a unique collaboration between occupational therapists from six different European countries and is the first pan-European occupational therapy textbook. I am proud to have been a part of this collaboration.

SECTION 1

INTRODUCTION

Chapter 1: The ENOTHE Terminology Project

Chapter 2: The Language of Occupational Therapy

Chapter 3: The Conceptual Framework

This book defines key occupational therapy terms and discusses how they work together. It also considers how the professional meaning of words relates to their common usage. Most words have more than one meaning. There is usually a common meaning, which is understood by the majority of people within a linguistic, cultural and social group, and there may also be a specialized meaning that is used within a discipline or professional group. Occupational therapists do not use terms that are unique to the profession; we take ordinary words and give them specialized meanings. This means that occupational therapists have to think carefully about how our clients understand the language we use and select the words that will best communicate our meanings.

The book is in three parts. The three chapters in Section 1 give the background to the ENOTHE terminology project and introduce the European conceptual framework for occupational therapy. In Section 2, Chapters 4 to 11 describe in detail the eight clusters of concepts that make up the conceptual framework. This description is from the perspective of the person performing the activity. The three chapters in Section 3 offer the perspective of the occupational therapist on understanding, measuring and facilitating the actions of her clients.

The three chapters in this first section introduce the European conceptual framework for occupational therapy. Chapter 1 describes the European Network of Occupational Therapy in Higher Education (ENOTHE) terminology project, which produced the conceptual framework. Chapter 2 discusses occupational therapy epistemology and terminology, offering an explanation of the difficulties that occupational therapists have with their professional vocabulary. Chapter 3 outlines the conceptual framework and explains its special characteristics.

It is not necessary to read the book in the order in which it has been written. A practitioner may, for example, prefer to start with Chapter 14, which describes how the conceptual framework can be used as a guide for practice, and then refer back to the chapters in Section 2 for more detailed discussion of specific terms. A student may begin at Chapter 3, which outlines the conceptual framework. An occupational therapy teacher may use individual chapters as the basis for tuition and discussion on particular concepts.

CHAPTER 1

THE ENOTHE TERMINOLOGY PROJECT

INTRODUCTION

This book is the outcome of a unique collaboration between occupational therapists from six European countries speaking six different languages. It presents a conceptual framework that has been constructed from the key terms used by occupational therapists to describe and explain their work. This framework describes the relationships between a set of clearly defined terms and represents a consensus on the meaning of, and relationships between, the concepts and theories underpinning occupational therapy practice throughout Europe. The framework is intended to provide a coherent foundation for the development of occupational therapy theory.

The concepts and their definitions have been translated into all the languages of the terminology working group, so that the conceptual framework is both relevant and accessible to occupational therapists working across Europe.

How the chapter is organized

This chapter gives the background to the European Network of Occupational Therapy in Higher Education (ENOTHE) terminology project and describes the method used to develop a European terminology for occupational therapy. It finishes with a brief explanation of how the terms have been organized into two sections. Twenty-five terms refer to the performer's experience of occupation, and these have been organized into the European conceptual framework for occupational therapy. The remaining five terms refer to the observer perspective of the therapist; these terms explain how occupational therapists use their understanding of occupation to design and implement therapeutic interventions with their clients.

THE TERMINOLOGY WORKING GROUP

The European Network of Occupational Therapy in Higher Education was founded in 1995 on the initiative of the Council of Occupational Therapists for European Countries (COTEC). It is a thematic network funded by the European Socrates/Erasmus programme for the purpose of building cooperation between higher educational institutions, other academic organizations and professional bodies. ENOTHE supports a variety of projects, all contributing to the development of a European dimension to occupational therapy education.

In 2000, ENOTHE identified that two of the biggest barriers to the harmonization of professional education across Europe were the lack of uniformity in occupational therapy terminology and the language differences between member countries and member institutions. In order for students and staff moving between universities to be able to communicate effectively, they need to know that the words they use represent the same concepts in different countries. Therefore, a common terminology is a necessary aspect of harmonizing occupational therapy education across Europe. One of the objectives set for the years 2001–2004 was to create a uniform terminology and make it accessible to non-English-speaking occupational therapists and lecturers by producing a glossary of occupational therapy terms in four languages. In order for this objective to be achieved, delegates at the ENOTHE annual conference in 2001 were invited to volunteer to form a working group for the purpose of initiating and carrying out the terminology project.

The first group of volunteers consisted of five people, representing five languages: English, French, German, Greek and Portuguese. Since 2001, the membership of the group has changed several times (Box 1.1). At the time when the current piece of work was carried out, the group consisted of six members, from Austria, Belgium, Portugal, Spain, Switzerland and the United Kingdom. These occupational therapists represent six languages: Dutch, English, French, German, Portuguese and Spanish, with

English adopted as the working language of the group. The advantages of using English were that most of the occupational therapy literature, at the beginning of the twenty-first century, was written in English and that all members of the group spoke English fluently.

Box 1.1: Membership of the ENOTHE terminology project group 2001–2008

Miguel Brea Rivero (2002–2008) Facultad de Ciencias de la Salud, Universidad Rey Juan Carlos, Madrid, Spain.

Jennifer Creek (2003–2008) Freelance practitioner, United Kingdom.

Joaquim Faias (2001–2008) Escola Superior de Tecnologia da Saúde do Porto, Portugal.

Andreas Fisher (2001–2002) Fachhochschule Osnabruck, Institut für Gesundheitsberufe, Germany.

Maria Hoppe (2001–2002) Individual contributor to ENOTHE, Krumpendorf, Austria.

Sarah Kantartzis (2001–2006) Technological Educational Institution of Athens, Greece. (Link person to the ENOTHE Board between 2003 and 2006.)

Sylvie Meyer (2002–2008) HES-SO Haute école de travail social et de la santé, Switzerland.

Martine Paban (2001–2002) Institut de Formation en Ergothérapie, Montpellier, France.

Hilde Pitteljon (2005–2008) Katholieke Hogeschool Brugge-Oostende, Belgium.

Linda Renton Queen Margaret University College, Edinburgh, United Kingdom. (Link person to the ENOTHE Board between 2001 and 2003.)

Ann de Ryck (2002–2004) Artevelde Hogeschool, Gent, Belgium.

Johanna Stadler-Grillmaier (2002–2008) Akademie für Ergotherapie, Vienna, Austria.

Liliya Todorova (Link person to the ENOTHE Board between 2006 and 2008.)

HOW THE TERMINOLOGY WAS DEVELOPED

From 2002 to 2008, the ENOTHE terminology group met two to three times a year to work on the project. In between face-to-face meetings, group members continued to work in their own countries and maintain regular email contact.

The group developed a method for producing definitions of key occupational therapy terms and a protocol for translating each definition into the languages of all the group members. There were four stages to this process:

1. selecting terms to define

2. collecting existing definitions of terms

3. constructing consensus definitions

4. translating the new definitions into the languages of the group.

Stage 1: Selecting terms

Early in the lifetime of the group, members agreed to define only core occupational therapy terms and not more general terms such as model, frame of reference and reasoning. The group began by choosing five terms that they felt represented core concepts in occupational therapy: *activity, function, occupation, occupational performance* and *occupational therapy*. The relationship between terms and concepts is discussed in more depth in Chapter 3. Once work on the definitions had started, members of the group took the decision that it was not necessary to define occupational therapy because each country already had its own definition. The World Federation of Occupational Therapists (WFOT) lists the definitions of occupational therapy used by member countries on its website (www.wfot. org./office_files/DEFINITIONS%20-%20DRAFT8%202007(2).pdf).

The terminology group therefore began its work by producing consensus definitions of four terms: *activity, function, occupation* and *occupational performance*. Once these definitions had been agreed, seven new terms were selected: *task, skill, occupational performance component, environment, role, occupational performance area* and *ability*. The process continued in this way for the six years of the project, with group members constructing definitions of selected terms and then identifying more key terms to work on. A total of 30 terms was selected over the course of the project, and these are listed in Box 1.2.

Stage 2: Collecting existing definitions of terms

The group decided to use existing definitions of key terms from the occupational therapy literature as a basis for constructing consensus definitions. Their search strategy was pragmatic rather than systematic, with group members searching textbooks and journal articles within their own institutions to identify existing definitions. Literature from national occupational therapy associations, the World Health Organization and the World Federation of Occupational Therapists was also searched.

Each group member looked at literature both in English and in her or his own language. Original definitions in languages other than English were translated into English for the purposes of the project. Definitions that were originally written in English and had been translated into other languages were not used. For some terms, such as *occupation*, many definitions were found but for others, such as *dependence*, there were few existing occupational therapy definitions.

All the definitions collected from the occupational therapy literature were collated on spreadsheets so that they could be analysed and compared.

Box 1.2: Terms selected for definition

Ability	Motivation
Activity	Occupation
Activity analysis	Occupational mapping
Activity performance	Occupational performance
Assessment	Occupational performance areas
Autonomy	Occupational performance components
Context	
Dependence	Participation
Engagement	Role
Environment	Routine
Evaluation	Setting
Function	Skill
Habit	Task
Independence	Task analysis
Interdependence	Task performance
	Volition

Stage 3: Constructing consensus definitions

Once existing definitions of a term had been collated, the next task was to analyse them in order to identify the elements contained within each definition. For example, one of the definitions taken from the literature was Kielhofner's (2002, p.117) definition of *skill*: 'observable, goal-directed actions that a person uses while performing'. The elements that make up this definition are:

- observable

- goal-directed

- actions

- used while performing.

For each term, the elements taken from all definitions found in the literature were collated to produce a comprehensive list. For example, the list of elements found in definitions of *skill* can be seen in Box 1.3.

Once the list of elements for a term was complete, the group constructed a consensus definition of the term using elements from the list. A consensus definition is one that is in accordance with the meanings of the majority of the original definitions of the term and that everyone in the working group could agree on. For example, the ENOTHE definition of *skill* was constructed from the elements of ability, practice and successful occupational performance, which became: 'an ability developed through practice which enables effective occupational performance'.

Part of the process of constructing consensus definitions was to consider how each term related to other, similar terms, so that all the definitions would work together. For example, it was necessary to think carefully about how the concepts of *skill* and *ability* relate to each other, what elements are common to both and how they differ.

Box 1.3: Elements found in occupational therapy definitions of *skill*

- features of what one does
- a vital component of occupation
- components
- categories
- in doing something
- required for performance
- required for successful performance
- required for the effective performance of a task or subtask
- smoothly integrated and sequenced, competent performance
- operating in performance
- used while performing
- understood in terms of performance
- performance of roles that are assumed by individuals in their lives
- the performance of various forms of purposeful behaviour
- activity and/or behaviour
- actions
- connect with the routines of their culture
- a specific ability or integrated set of abilities e.g. motor, sensory, cognitive or perceptual
- practised ability
- explained by the presence of various underlying general abilities
- the abilities that a person has
- the ability to put skill components together
- ability to construct an activity pattern
- appropriate sequencing
- an essential capacity of human beings
- learned and practised to a standard
- learned behaviours

Box 1.3: Elements found in occupational therapy definitions of *skill (continued)*

- learned

- level of proficiency

- goal-directed

- enables persons to achieve their purposes

- functional purposes

- match a model

- means of human adaptation

- product of human adaptation

- adaptation to the challenges of the environment

- understood in terms of self-perception

- related to observable elements of action

- observable

- in the context and environment

At this stage of the process, it was helpful to consider how the terms themselves would translate into the other languages of the group. In some languages, more than one word can be substituted for the English term: for example, *occupation* can be translated into German as *Handlungen, Betätigungen* and *Tätigkeiten*. The boundaries between concepts are not necessarily the same in different languages, which helped the group to see more clearly what those boundaries are in English. It was also important, when constructing the English definitions, to take into account how those definitions could be translated into other languages.

The consensus definitions of the selected terms are shown in Box 1.4. Two of the terms, *function* and *task*, are used by occupational therapists with two distinct meanings and have each been given two definitions. The definitions of *occupational performance, activity performance* and *task performance* are the same, except for the words occupations/activities/tasks.

Box 1.4: The consensus definitions

Ability: A personal characteristic that supports occupational performance.

Activity: A structured series of actions or tasks that contribute to occupations.

Activity analysis: Breaking up an activity into the components that influence how it is chosen, organized and carried out in interaction with the environment.

Assessment: A process of collecting, analysing and interpreting information about people's functions and environments, using observation, testing and measurement, in order to make intervention decisions and to monitor changes.

Autonomy: The freedom to make choices based on consideration of internal and external circumstances and to act on those choices.

Context: The relationships between the environment, personal factors and events that influence the meaning of a task, activity or occupation for the performer.

Dependence: The condition of needing support in order to be able to perform everyday activities to a satisfactory level.

Engagement: A sense of involvement, choice, positive meaning and commitment while performing an occupation or activity.

Environment: External physical, sociocultural and temporal factors that demand and shape occupational performance.

Evaluation: The process of obtaining, interpreting and appraising information (about occupational performance) in order to prioritize problems and needs, to plan and modify interventions and to judge the worth of interventions.

Function 1: The underlying physical and psychological components that support occupational performance.

Function 2: The capacity to use occupational performance components to carry out a task, activity or occupation.

Habit: A performance pattern in daily life, acquired by frequent repetition, that does not require attention and allows efficient function.

Independence: The condition of being able to perform everyday activities to a satisfactory level.

Interdependence: The condition of mutual dependence and influence between members of a social group.

Motivation: A drive that directs a person's actions towards meeting needs.

Occupation: A group of activities that has personal and sociocultural meaning, is named within a culture and supports participation in society. Occupations can be categorized as self-care, productivity and/or leisure.

Occupational/activity/task performance: Choosing, organizing and carrying out occupations/activities/tasks in interaction with the environment.

Box 1.4: The consensus definitions *(continued)*

Occupational mapping: A collaborative process between the therapist and client through which the person's subjective experience of occupation can be explored.

Occupational performance areas: Categories of tasks, activities and occupations that are typically part of daily life. They are usually called self-care, productivity and leisure.

Occupational performance components: Abilities and skills that enable and affect engagement in tasks, activities and occupations. These can be categorized, for example, as physical, cognitive, psychosocial and affective.

Participation: Involvement in life situations through activity within a social context.

Role: Social and cultural norms and expectations of occupational performance that are associated with the individual's social and personal identity.

Routine: An established and predictable sequence of tasks.

Setting: The immediate surroundings that influence task, activity or occupational performance.

Skill: An ability developed through practice which enables effective occupational performance.

Task: A series of structured steps (actions and/or thoughts) intended to accomplish a specific goal. This goal could either be:

1.   the performance of an activity

2.   a piece of work the individual is expected to do.

Task analysis: Breaking up an activity into its task sequence.

Volition: The ability to choose to do or continue to do something, together with an awareness that the performance of the activity is voluntary.

The terminology group was unable to find a definition of *occupational analysis* in the literature, although the term is sometimes used by occupational therapists (for example, Persson *et al.* 2001). After much discussion, group members decided to use the term *occupational mapping* as an alternative, because it seemed a more appropriate label for the concept they were trying to define. No definitions of the term were found so the definition was constructed from the description of occupational mapping given in Morel-Bracq *et al.* (2008).

INFLUENCE OF THE ICF

In the development of the European terminology, project group members took account of the ICF: *International Classification of Functioning, Disability and Health* (World Health Organization 2001). This system of classification for health-related terms was designed 'to provide a uniform and standard language and framework for the description of health and health-related states' (p.3) and is becoming the common language for health care professionals worldwide. The ICF was not developed to replace the language of individual professions but to complement it. It has been widely explored and used by occupational therapists (Stewart 2007) and has been found to be broadly compatible with occupational therapy theories (Farrell *et al.* 2007).

During the development of the consensus definitions, the project group took care to ensure that the ENOTHE terminology is consistent with the language of the ICF. For example, the definitions of *function*, *activity*, *participation* and *environment* in the European conceptual framework are all compatible with the definitions in the ICF. However, the ICF classification and language cannot replace any conceptual framework or model for occupational therapy because that would bring about the loss of some of the richness and complexity of meaning that occupational therapists give to the words they use. For example, the word *function*, for an occupational therapist, means the capacity to use occupational performance components to carry out a task, activity or occupation: we might talk about self-care functions or about having a good level of function in activities of daily life. In the ICF, the word is given a much narrower meaning: 'the physiological functions of body systems' (World Health Organization 2001, p.10): for example, we might say that someone has poor cognitive function. The ICF definition highlighted for the group that occupational therapists use the term *function* in both senses: meaning either how well a person can do the things he wants to do, needs to do or is expected to do in daily life or the body systems themselves. To accommodate these two meanings, *function* has been given two definitions in the conceptual framework.

The other word that is used in two distinct senses by occupational therapists is *task*, which can mean both the steps intended to accomplish the performance of an activity and a piece of work that the individual is expected to do. The word *task* has also been given two definitions in the conceptual framework.

Stage 4: Translating the terms and definitions

Once each consensus definition had been agreed, it was translated into the languages of the working group by the members. First, each group member had to select the most appropriate word in her or his language to represent the concept. The group found that, in some cases, they could agree on a consensus definition of a concept but could not find a word to represent it that was agreed by colleagues in their own country. The definition could then be used to explain the meaning of several different words and therapists could choose which one to use.

Validation of the translations was achieved by consulting a panel of experts in each country, drawn from national associations, educational institutions and clinical settings. These experts were asked to comment on the grammatical construction and elegance of the translations, not on the content of definitions. As the definitions and translations were finished, they were put on the ENOTHE website (www.enothe.hva.nl).

In order for additional languages to be included in the project, the group designed a protocol for the process of translation that would ensure a consistently high quality. This process includes identifying occupational therapy and language experts who are recognized by the ENOTHE Board, approving the translation by national associations or ENOTHE member schools and providing a back translation if required by the ENOTHE board.

Other terms

The ENOTHE Board requested that the terminology group define some of the new terms that have come into use by occupational therapists in recent years, such as *occupational balance* and *occupational justice*. New terms are coined or adopted to represent new concepts that underpin theoretical developments in occupational therapy. The proliferation of new terms over the past few years illustrates the rapid expansion of the occupational therapy theory base, which has been driven by changes in modes of service delivery, advances in the discipline of occupational science and an increasing political awareness within the profession.

Some of these new terms have come into use so recently that there is not yet a substantial body of literature from which consensus definitions can be constructed. The terminology working group took the decision that, as an interim measure, an existing definition of each term would be selected from the occupational therapy literature for use within the terminology project. These nine terms and their definitions are shown in Box 1.5.

Box 1.5: Selected definitions of new terms

Client-centred practice: Collaborative and partnership approaches used in enabling occupation with clients who may be individuals, groups, agencies, governments, corporations or others; client-centred occupational therapists demonstrate respect for clients, involve clients in decision making, advocate with and for clients' needs, and otherwise recognize clients' experience and knowledge. (Townsend *et al.* 2002, p.180)

Enablement: [The process of creating opportunities] to participate in life's tasks and occupations irrespective of physical or mental impairment or environmental challenges. (Christiansen and Townsend 2004, p.276)

Occupational alienation: A sense that one's occupations are meaningless and unfulfilling, typically associated with feelings of powerlessness to alter the situation. (Hagedorn 2001, p.166)

Occupational apartheid: [A state resulting] from political constraints which may extend to encompass all aspects of daily living and human occupation through legal, economic, social, and religious restrictions, and can be found as a consequence of chronic poverty and inequality. (Kronenberg and Pollard 2005, p.66)

Occupational balance: Managing [occupation] in a way that is personally fulfilling...and meets role demands... Each person has an individual balance schema that suits his or her health. (Reed and Sanderson 1999, p.99)

Occupational deprivation: A state of prolonged preclusion from engagement in occupations of necessity or meaning due to factors outside the control of an individual, such as through geographic isolation, incarceration or disability. (Christiansen and Townsend 2004, p.278)

Occupational imbalance: Inability to manage occupations in a way that is personally fulfilling and meets role demands, leading to health and quality of life being compromized. (Christiansen and Townsend 2004, p.278; Reed and Sanderson 1999, p.99)

Occupational justice: A critical perspective of social structures that promotes social, political, and economic changes to enable people to meet their occupational potential and experience well-being [and full citizenship]. (Crepeau, Cohn and Schell 2003, p.1031)

Occupational science: Academic discipline of the social sciences aimed at producing a body of knowledge on occupation through theory generation, and systematic, disciplined methods of inquiry. (Crepeau, Cohn and Schell 2003, p.1031)

HOW THE TERMS HAVE BEEN ORGANIZED

When occupational therapists think about their clients' occupations, they do so from two perspectives: their own perspective as an observer and the client's perspective as a performer. As group members explored the 30 concepts defined in the terminology project, they realized that some terms refer to the performer's experience of occupation and some refer to the observer's view of what the performer is doing.

The 25 terms that refer to aspects of the performer's experience are: ability, activity, activity performance, autonomy, context, dependence, engagement, environment, function, habit, independence, interdependence, motivation, occupation, occupational performance, occupational performance areas, occupational performance components, participation, role, routine, setting, skill, task, task performance and volition. These terms have been organized into the European conceptual framework for occupational therapy, which is described in the second section of this book. The framework provides a web of concepts that describe and explain how a person experiences occupation.

The five terms that refer to the observer's perspective are: activity analysis, assessment, evaluation, occupational mapping and task analysis. These terms are explored in the last section of the book. Together, these five terms explain how the therapist uses her or his understanding of occupation, of occupational performance and of a person's experience of occupation to design and implement therapeutic interventions.

SUMMARY

This chapter began by describing how the ENOTHE terminology project came into being. It then outlined the method used to develop a European terminology for occupational therapy and the method of translating the English terms and definitions into other languages. The chapter finished with an explanation of the difference between the performer's and observer's perspectives on occupation. The performer's perspective is represented by the 25 terms in the European conceptual framework for occupational therapy. The observer's perspective is represented by five terms that occupational therapists use to refer to the means by which they design and implement therapeutic interventions with their clients.

The next chapter explores occupational therapy language and epistemology.

REFERENCES

Christiansen, C.H. and Townsend, E.A. (2004) *Introduction to Occupation: The Art and Science of Living*. Upper Saddle River, NJ: Prentice Hall.

Crepeau, E.B., Cohn, E.S. and Schell, B.A.B. (eds) (2003) *Willard & Spackman's Occupational Therapy, Tenth Edition*. Philadelphia, PA: Lippincott Williams & Wilkins.

Farrell, J., Anderson, S., Hewitt, K., Livingston, M.H. and Stewart, D. (2007) 'A survey of occupational therapists in Canada about their knowledge and use of the ICF.' *Canadian Journal of Occupational Therapy 74 (ICF Special Issue)*, 221–232.

Hagedorn, R. (2001) *Foundations for Practice in Occupational Therapy, Third Edition*. Edinburgh: Churchill Livingstone.

Kielhofner, G. (2002) *Model of Human Occupation: Theory and Application, Third Edition*. Baltimore, MD: Lippincott Williams & Wilkins.

Kronenberg, F. and Pollard, N. (2005) 'Overcoming occupational apartheid: a preliminary exploration of the political nature of occupational therapy.' In F. Kroneneberg, S.S. Algado and N. Pollard (eds) *Occupational Therapy without Borders: Learning from the Spirit of Survivors*. Edinburgh: Elsevier.

Morel-Bracq, M., Burgess-Morris, K., Cirtautas, A., Market, M., May, G. and Randlov, B. (2008) *Teaching and Learning: Activity Analysis and Occupational Mapping*. Amsterdam: ENOTHE.

Persson, D., Erlandsson, L.K., Eklund, M. and Iwarsson, S. (2001) 'Value dimensions: meaning and complexity in human occupation – a tentative structure for analysis.' *Scandinavian Journal of Occupational Therapy 8*, 7–18.

Reed, K.L. and Sanderson, S.N. (1999) *Concepts of Occupational Therapy. Fourth Edition*. Philadelphia, PA: Lippincott Williams & Wilkins.

Stewart, D. (2007) 'Editorial.' *Canadian Journal of Occupational Therapy 74 (ICF Special Issue)*, 217–218.

Townsend, E., Stanton, S., Law, M., Polatajkon, H and Baptiste, S. (2002) *Enabling Occupation: An Occupational Therapy Perspective*. Revised edition. Ottawa: Canadian Association of Occupational Therapists.

World Health Organization (2001) *International Classification of Functioning, Disability and Health*. Geneva: World Health Organization.

CHAPTER 2

THE LANGUAGE OF OCCUPATIONAL THERAPY

INTRODUCTION

Chapter 1 described the background to the European Network of Occupational Therapy in Higher Education (ENOTHE) terminology project and the method used to develop a European terminology for occupational therapy. This chapter discusses the difficulties that occupational therapists have had in finding a language to express their professional identity and practice.

Language is a tool that people use both to communicate about what they do and to think about what they do. The language that we use for both these purposes is important because it not only shapes how other people see our actions but can also influence how we feel about what we are doing. The words that a person selects to describe his or her actions are not neutral but have an impact on how he or she thinks and feels. For example, if I think of cooking the evening meal as an unwelcome chore, I am likely to experience the meal preparation as dull and boring, providing little opportunity for me to express my individuality. On the other hand, if I think of cooking the evening meal as a creative act, I am likely to approach the task with interest and to feel engaged in what I am doing.

Having a coherent professional vocabulary is important to occupational therapists for three reasons: for thinking clearly and logically about how activity can be employed as a therapeutic medium for enhancing occupational performance; for communicating precisely with colleagues for the purposes of teaching, research and sharing good practice; and for explaining the purpose and process of occupational therapy to clients, service commissioners, managers, colleagues from other disciplines and the general public.

How the chapter is organized

The chapter begins with an account of the difficulties that occupational therapists have had in finding a common language to describe what they do. It argues that words represent concepts and that concepts shape how we think and perceive, therefore, using different words can change the way that we see the world. Occupational therapy is described as a profession with two ways of seeing the world, or two competing epistemologies: pragmatism and structuralism. However, the profession is currently undergoing an epistemological transformation, as it progresses from organizing its knowledge base on a structuralist model to acknowledging that a more dynamic way of knowing and thinking is needed to encompass the complexity of occupation and health.

OCCUPATIONAL THERAPISTS' PROBLEM WITH LANGUAGE

Despite recognizing the importance of professional language, occupational therapists seem to have difficulty finding appropriate words with which to think about and express the nature and purpose of their practice. Occupational therapy theorists and writers have made many attempts to reach agreement on the meaning of key concepts and the relationships between them, but this has not yet been achieved (College of Occupational Therapists 2004; Golledge 1998; Hagedorn 2000; Katz and Sachs 1991).

Occupational therapists in Europe have an additional problem: that of the many languages spoken across the continent. Not only does the profession need to agree on the meaning of key concepts, such as *occupation* and *function*, in English, but there also has to be agreement on these meanings in Finnish, Lithuanian, French, Greek and all the other languages spoken across Europe. Reaching agreement on the precise meaning of key occupational therapy terms in all the main European languages would make it possible to communicate more effectively for the purpose of collaboration in practice, teaching, research and theory development, as shown in Example 2.1.

Example 2.1: Reaching agreement on the meaning of key terms

A number of occupational therapists working in several European countries decided to apply for joint funding to do a multi-site study of the impact of physical activity on the level of independence of older people living at home. In order to be sure that they were all studying the same thing, they had to agree exactly what they meant by *activity* and *independence*.

Occupational therapy practitioners, educators, managers, researchers and scholars want to be able to talk and write about their work in language that is understood by their audiences yet, more than 80 years after the first occupational therapist was employed in the UK (Paterson 2002), the profession still worries that people in general have not heard of occupational therapy (Gillibrand, Potter and Spittle 2007) and that the commissioners of services do not understand the value of their work (OTN 2007). Several reasons can be identified for this continuing problem.

Occupational therapy authors regularly introduce their own definitions of key professional words, such as *occupation* and *activity*, or avoid defining the terms altogether, leaving readers to make up their own minds about what is meant. This makes it impossible to compare the work of different writers. For example, a review of evidence for a relationship between what people do and their health (Creek and Hughes 2008) found papers that used either the term *activity* or the term *occupation*, or both. In some papers written by occupational therapists, occupation and activity appeared to mean the same thing (Iwarsson *et al.* 1998; Mozley 2001), other papers referred to specific areas of occupation, such as leisure (Passmore 2003), while non-occupational therapy authors used the term activity rather than occupation (Friedland *et al.* 2001; Glass *et al.* 1999; Reynolds 2000), unless they used the latter term to mean employment (O'Brien 1981).

Christiansen and Townsend (2004) pointed out that the everyday meanings of words are not precise enough for the purposes of comparison or analysis. For example, when students are learning how to do task analysis and activity analysis, they need to understand exactly what is meant by *task* and *activity* and what the relationship is between these two concepts. If the educator is not able to communicate the precise meanings of these terms, students will be confused about what they are trying to learn.

Another factor contributing to conceptual confusion within occupational therapy is the uncritical transfer of terms, and the concepts they represent, from one culture to another. Many theories and models developed by occupational therapists in North America have been adopted in other English-speaking countries without critical appraisal of their cultural relevance. Non-English-speaking occupational therapists have also translated key terms from English into their own languages without fully understanding the concepts that the words represent. Hooper (2006) criticized this practice as a failure to examine the epistemology represented by terminology.

EPISTEMOLOGY AND OCCUPATIONAL THERAPY

Words are the labels given to concepts. For example, the concepts that make up the knowledge base of occupational therapy are labelled *occupation, activity, function,* and so on. Learning a new subject always entails learning a new vocabulary with which to refer to the concepts that underpin the topic.

The words that we use point to an underlying frame of reference, or way of knowing, which shapes how we think about what we see. This means that when we change our frame of reference we find ourselves using different words, as shown in Example 2.2.

Example 2.2: The language of frames of reference

An occupational therapist working within a psychodynamic frame of reference might describe her client's dysfunction in terms of immature object relations or weak ego strength. If she switches to using a human developmental perspective, she might describe the same deficits as developmental delay or maladaptive skills development.

The same word can mean different things depending on both the frame of reference adopted and the context in which it is used, as illustrated by Example 2.3.

Example 2.3: Language and context

An occupational therapist discussing the influence of the environment in which therapy takes place uses the word *setting* to mean 'the context of occupational therapy intervention' (Thompson 1990, p.115). When she is talking about making jewellery with her clients, she uses the word *setting* to mean the frame in which a stone is set.

An American occupational therapist, Hooper (2006), wrote of the importance of understanding *how* we know, not just *what* we know; of examining the ways that we take in and make sense of experience, that is, our epistemology. Hooper claimed that our chosen epistemology 'functions as a screen through which we filter the experiences we consider important from those we do not' (p.16). However, most of the time, people are not aware that they have a particular way of knowing, or that there are alternative perspectives.

Two distinct epistemologies have been identified within occupational therapy: pragmatism and structuralism. Pragmatism is a philosophy which stresses the relationship between theory and action (Audi 1999): it has been described as 'the philosophy of "common sense", problem solving, activity, and adaptation' (Breines 1986, p.56). In contrast, structuralism is concerned with the underlying structures that are shared by phenomena, rather than with individual difference and context-dependent action (Hooper and Wood 2002). Knowledge is seen as 'objectively fixed, theoretically neutral, context free, universal, and derived from external authority' (p.46).

Each of these two ways of knowing leads to a different way of conceptualizing the goals of occupational therapy and, hence, to divergent approaches to practice. This duality has led to what the American anthropologist Cheryl Mattingly (1994a, p.37) called a 'two-body practice'.

The first focus of occupational therapy practice, arising from a structuralist epistemology, is the 'functional problems that fall nicely within biomedicine (treating physical injuries with specific treatment techniques)' (Mattingly 1994a, p.37). Mattingly called this a focus on 'the body as machine' (p.37). The occupational therapist who takes a structuralist perspective 'work[s] toward goals that relate to the physiological problems of dysfunction (thus being disease- or injury-focused)' (p.38).

The second focus of occupational therapists' two-body practice, arising from their pragmatist philosophy, is 'the lived body' (Mattingly 1994b, p.64). The occupational therapist who works with the lived body takes a pragmatic approach to the client, locating him within real-life situations and framing his problems in terms of his interactions with his physical and social environments. She sees that illness or disability do not just affect the body and mind but interrupt people's whole lives.

Hooper (2006) carried out an epistemological analysis of occupational therapy's history over nine decades and concluded that occupational therapy is currently undergoing an epistemological transformation. She claimed that new ways of knowing 'are emerging in, and demanded by,' (p.20) occupational therapy practice as we move towards more dynamic, complex ways of conceptualizing occupation and health.

Paradigm shift in occupational therapy

At the beginning of the twentieth century, the first occupational therapists worked under the direction of doctors, having no theory base to inform their practice:

> Early occupational therapists had a moral philosophy and a moral imperative to train more practitioners but no knowledge base of their own with which to educate them or much of any status or expertise with which to argue for particular educational practices. (Hooper and Wood 2002, p.46)

From the early 1960s onwards, beginning in North America, occupational therapists began to develop theories that would describe and guide their practice, building a substantial body of knowledge and developing a variety of approaches for translating that knowledge into action. Some of the occupational therapy knowledge base was adopted from other disciplines, such as medicine and psychology, while some was developed within the profession. The profession's body of knowledge has continued to grow and develop.

In the 1960s, an American occupational therapy educator, Mary Reilly, suggested that the profession should develop a general theory of occupational therapy, which synthesized biological, psychological and social sciences, rather than using different theories in different fields of practice. She advocated the use of general systems theory as an organizing framework for the knowledge base (Reilly 1974).

General systems theory is a structuralist way of understanding the relationships between elements in the material world, such as rocks, leaves, trees, cats and people. It is hierarchical in organization, categorizing elements at different levels of complexity, each level subordinate to the ones above and incorporating the ones below. For example, atoms are made of protons and electrons, molecules are made of atoms, cells are made of molecules, men are made of cells and social organizations are made of men (Boulding 1968).

Using general systems theory as an organizing framework, occupational therapists view the relationships between key concepts as fixed and hierarchical. For example, in 2004, a group of Canadian occupational therapists produced a taxonomy of seven terms referring to occupational performance: occupational grouping, occupation, activity, task, action, movement pattern and voluntary movement. Occupational grouping is the highest and voluntary movement the lowest level of taxonomy.

For several decades, general systems theory provided occupational therapy with hierarchical structures that were used to organize the knowledge generated by research and scholarly activity. Eventually, however, this way of seeing the world was challenged: by demographic changes, leading to new patterns of need; by theoretical influences, and by research findings. It became increasingly obvious that general systems theory was no longer adequate to explain how the elements of occupational therapy practice relate to each other.

In the twenty-first century, the language of complexity and dynamic systems theory is being used increasingly in the occupational therapy literature (Creek 2003; Gray, Kennedy and Zemke 1996; Hooper 2006; Whiteford, Klomp and Wright-St Clair 2005), replacing the language of structuralism. This suggests a fundamental change in the epistemology of occupational therapy, from organizing concepts into hierarchies to seeing the relationships between concepts as fluid and dynamic.

The complexity of occupational therapy theory and practice comes, in part, from the large number of factors that the therapist must be aware of when working with the lived body. Not only does the therapist have to take into account her or his own beliefs, values, goals, knowledge, skills, tools, methods, culture, language and experience, and the client's history, experience, language, context, thoughts, beliefs, values, aspirations, needs, problems, goals, interests, occupations, relationships, potentials, skills and abilities, but she or he also has to adapt to external influences, including the working environment, the evidence base for practice, local and national policies and the wider social and cultural environments in which therapy takes place (Creek 2003).

A fuller explanation of complexity theory, and of how it has informed the development of the European conceptual framework for occupational therapy, is given in Chapter 3.

SUMMARY

This chapter presented a brief account of the difficulties that occupational therapists have had in finding a common language to describe what they do. It described occupational therapy as a profession with two competing epistemologies: pragmatism and structuralism. Occupational therapy is currently undergoing an epistemological transformation, as it progresses from using general systems theory as the organizing framework for theory to acknowledging that the complexity of the relationship between occupation and health demands a more dynamic way of knowing and thinking. These ideas are dealt with in more depth in the next chapter.

REFERENCES

Audi, R. (ed.) (1999) *The Cambridge Dictionary of Philosophy, Second Edition.* Cambridge: Cambridge University Press.

Boulding, K.E. (1968) 'General systems theory – the skeleton of science.' In W. Buckley (ed.) *Modern Systems Research for the Behavioural Scientist.* Chicago, IL: Aldine.

Breines, E. (1986) *Origins and Adaptations: A Philosophy of Practice.* Lebanon, NJ: Geri-Rehab Inc.

Christiansen, C.H. and Townsend, E.A. (2004) 'An introduction to occupation.' In C. Christiansen and E.A. Townsend (eds) *Introduction to Occupation: The Art and Science of Living.* Upper Saddle River, NJ: Prentice Hall.

College of Occupational Therapists (2004) *Occupational Therapy Standard Terminology Project Report.* London: College of Occupational Therapists.

Creek, J. (2003) *Occupational Therapy Defined as a Complex Intervention.* London: College of Occupational Therapists.

Creek, J. and Hughes, A. (2008) 'Occupation and health: a review of selected literature.' *British Journal of Occupational Therapy 71*, 11, 456–468.

Friedland, R.P., Fritsch, T., Smyth, K.A., Koss, E., *et al.* (2001) 'Patients with Alzheimer's disease have reduced activities in midlife compared with healthy control-group members.' *Proceedings of the National Academy of Sciences 98*, 6, 3440–3445.

Gillibrand, K., Potter, N. and Spittle, A. (2007) 'OT...never heard of it.' *Occupational Therapy News 15*, 12, 38.

Glass, T.A., Mendes de Leon, C., Marottoli, R.A. and Berkman, L.F. (1999) 'Population based study of social and productive activities as predictors of survival among elderly Americans.' *British Medical Journal 319*, 478–483.

Golledge, J. (1998) 'Distinguishing between occupation, purposeful activity and activity, Part 1: review and explanation.' *British Journal of Occupational Therapy 61*, 3, 100–105.

Gray, J.M., Kennedy, B.L. and Zemke, R. (1996) 'Application of dynamic systems theory to occupation.' In R. Zemke and F. Clark (eds) *Occupational Science: The Evolving Discipline.* Philadelphia, PA: F.A. Davis.

Hagedorn, R. (2000) *Tools for Practice in Occupational Therapy: A Structured Approach to Core Skills and Processes.* Edinburgh: Churchill Livingstone.

Hooper, B. (2006) 'Epistemological transformation in occupational therapy: educational implications and challenges.' *OTJR: Occupation, Participation and Health 26*, 1, 15–24.

Hooper, B. and Wood, W. (2002) 'Pragmatism and structuralism in occupational therapy: the long conversation.' *American Journal of Occupational Therapy 56*, 1, 40–50.

Iwarsson, S., Isacsson, Å., Persson, D. and Scherstén, B. (1998) 'Occupation and survival: a 25-year follow-up study of an aging population.' *American Journal of Occupational Therapy 52*, 1, 65–70.

Katz, N. and Sachs, D. (1991) 'Meaning ascribed to major professional concepts: a comparison of occupational therapy students and practitioners in the United States and Israel.' *American Journal of Occupational Therapy 45*, 2, 137–145.

Mattingly, C. (1994a) 'Occupational therapy as a two-body practice: the body as machine.' In C. Mattingly and M.H. Fleming *Clinical Reasoning: Forms of Inquiry in a Therapeutic Practice.* Philadelphia, PA: F.A. Davis.

Mattingly, C. (1994b) 'Occupational therapy as a two-body practice: the lived body.' In C. Mattingly and M.H. Fleming *Clinical Reasoning: Forms of Inquiry in a Therapeutic Practice.* Philadelphia, PA: F.A. Davis.

Mozley, C.G. (2001) 'Exploring connections between occupation and mental health in care homes for older people.' *Journal of Occupational Science 8*, 3, 14–19.

O'Brien, G.E. (1981) 'Locus of control, previous occupation and satisfaction with retirement.' *Australian Journal of Psychology 33*, 3, 305–318.

OTN (2007) 'OT week is on the horizon: promoting the OT profession.' *Occupational Therapy News 15*, 9, 6.

Passmore, A. (2003) 'The occupation of leisure: three typologies and their influence on mental health in adolescence.' *OTJR: Occupation, Participation and Health 23*, 2, 76–83.

Paterson, C.F. (2002) 'A short history of occupational therapy in psychiatry.' In J. Creek (ed.) *Occupational Therapy and Mental Health, Third Edition.* Edinburgh: Churchill Livingstone.

Polatajko, H.J., Davis, J.A., Hobson, S.J.G., Landry, J.E., *et al.* (2004) 'Meeting the responsibility that comes with the privilege: introducing a taxonomic code for understanding occupation.' *Canadian Journal of Occupational Therapy 71*, 5, 261–264.

Reilly, M. (1974) 'An explanation of play.' In M. Reilly (ed.) *Play as Exploratory Learning: Studies of Curiosity Behaviour.* Beverly Hills, CA: Sage.

Reynolds, F. (2000) 'Managing depression through needlecraft creative activities: a qualitative study.' *The Arts in Psychotherapy 27*, 2, 107–114.

Thompson, B. (1990) 'Roles and settings.' In J. Creek (ed.) *Occupational Therapy and Mental Health: Principles, Skills and Practice.* Edinburgh: Churchill Livingstone.

Whiteford, G., Klomp, N. and Wright-St Clair, V. (2005) 'Complexity theory: understanding occupation, practice and context.' In G. Whiteford and V. Wright-St Clair (eds) *Occupation and Practice in Context.* Sydney: Elsevier.

CHAPTER 3

THE CONCEPTUAL FRAMEWORK

INTRODUCTION

Chapter 2 presented a brief account of the difficulties that occupational therapists have had in finding a common language to describe what they do, in part due to having adopted two competing epistemologies: pragmatism and structuralism. It was suggested that this dichotomy may be resolved by abandoning the use of general systems theory as an organizing framework for the profession's knowledge base, and moving towards a fuller acknowledgement of the complexity of occupational therapy theory and practice.

This chapter presents a conceptual framework for occupational therapy in Europe that has been constructed with complexity theory as the organizing principle. The conceptual framework is not a static framework, based on hierarchical relationships, but is a dynamic, complex structure that can accommodate the flexibility of expert occupational therapy practice.

What is a conceptual framework?

A conceptual framework is a structure made up of concepts displayed together in a way that shows how they relate to each other.

A concept is an idea of a class of objects or abstractions: for example, *activity* is a concept. The function of a concept is to enable the mind to point out, denote or attend to something (Dickoff, James and Wiedenbach

1968). We can only talk about a concept if we give it a name: 'the essential function of naming is the giving of a tag to enable reference...to, or communicating about, the factor' (*ibid.* p.420). If a concept is not named, we cannot think about it, talk about it or compare it with other concepts. For example, the concept of *occupational justice* did not exist for occupational therapists until the name was coined.

A framework is a structure made of parts that are joined together to act as a support or enclosure. We may think of a framework as a static form, such as the wooden frame of a house, but it can also be dynamic. For example, I can make my hands into a framework to hold a baby but they will not remain static: my fingers flex and move to accommodate the child's shape and movements.

How the chapter is organized

This chapter provides an introduction to the European conceptual framework: a more detailed description can be found in Chapters 4 to 11. The chapter begins with a brief account of how the framework was developed, using the principles of complexity theory as a guide. A short account of complexity theory is offered, with an explanation of how it informed the construction of the framework. The last section of the chapter gives an overview of the conceptual framework and describes its key characteristics: the observer and performer perspectives; the clusters; the internal and external worlds; the dynamic nature of relationships between the terms, and the dimensions.

DEVELOPING THE CONCEPTUAL FRAMEWORK

When the terminology group was first formed, members thought that their job was to select key occupational therapy terms, agree on how they should be defined in English and translate them into other European languages. However, as the group analysed existing definitions, extracted elements of meaning and sought to agree on the boundaries between terms, it became apparent that what they were doing was not simply constructing consensus definitions of words. Words represent concepts and the group were, in fact, exploring, analysing and interpreting key occupational therapy concepts and the relationships between them. The process of isolating and naming concepts provides the foundation for theory development.

In the 1960s, two American philosophers, Dickoff and James (1968), wrote about the nature and development of theory in a practice discipline, using nursing as their model. They suggested that a theory is 'a conceptual system or framework invented to some purpose' (p.198) and that the overriding purpose of theory for a practice discipline, such as occupational therapy, is to enable practitioners to predict the outcomes of their interventions: 'If I do this with my client, then this will follow'. They called this type of theory *situation-producing theory* or *prescriptive theory*. An example of situation-producing theory in occupational therapy is the model of creative ability, developed by Vona du Toit in South Africa (de Witt 2005) (see Box 3.1).

Box 3.1: The model of creative ability

Creative ability is 'a combination of motivation and action, which results in the formation of a product' (du Toit 1991, p.47). The model of creative ability identifies six levels of motivation and ten levels of action, from predestructive action to society-centred action. It gives the therapist a structure for deciding what actions to take with clients who are performing at the different levels. The client can be helped to move from one level to the next by the provision of appropriate support, structure and encouragement: this is called the therapist-directed phase of intervention. As the client's performance improves, he is able to perform at the higher level in optimal conditions: this is called the transitional phase. Eventually, the client is able to maintain his performance independently, in what is called the patient-directed phase.

Dickoff and James (1968) further suggested that situation-producing theory presupposes the existence of more elementary types of theory: *naming theory* and *situation-depicting theory*. The first level of theory, naming theory, is so basic that it is frequently overlooked:

> the first act of the thinking mind is to make for itself its conceptual atoms or ideas. These most primitive concepts tend to be ideas whose function is to allow the mind to point out, denote, or attend to conceptually a factor within the mind's consciousness... The verbalization of these primitive ideas is often called naming [and] the essential function of naming is the giving of a tag to enable reference back to, or the pointing to, or communicating about the factor. (Dickoff *et al.* 1968, p.420)

For example, in the model of creative ability, two of the key concepts are *creative response*, which is the positive attitude of the individual towards any opportunities he is offered, and *creative participation*, which is the process of being actively involved in the activities of everyday living (de Witt 2005).

If we do not have names for concepts, we cannot think about them, talk about them or compare them with other concepts. For example, occupational therapists could not discuss the concept of *occupational alienation* until it was given a name.

The second level of theory is situation-depicting theory, which looks at concepts not in isolation but in relation to each other. 'An illuminating way to think of such theories may be as depictions or descriptions...at a given moment in time' (Dickoff *et al.* 1968, p.421). For example, in the model of creative ability, the creative response is described as a necessary precursor to, and accompaniment of, creative participation (de Witt 2005). By describing these concepts in relation to each other, du Toit went beyond the level of naming theory to situation-depicting theory.

The terminology working group also found themselves going beyond naming and defining isolated terms when they realized that the boundaries between concepts are not always clear or fixed. This process of situation-depicting was enhanced by the multilingual nature of the group. Discussions about the meaning of terms in the different languages of group members helped to clarify the precise meaning of each word in English, its relationship to similar concepts, what meanings the terms had in common, what the differences were and where concepts overlapped.

Clarification of the meanings of terms and of the boundaries between them led to the terms being grouped into clusters of closely related terms that together represent aspects of occupational therapy theory. For example, *motivation, volition* and *engagement* are all terms used by occupational therapists to refer to the emotional energy that people put into their activities (Figure 3.1).

Once agreement had been reached on how the terms could be clustered, the terminology group then began to explore the relationships between clusters and to map them into a conceptual framework. In order to make sense of these relationships, to explain what type of relationships they were and to have a language for talking about them, the group needed to find an appropriate theory. Group members were aware of increasing references to complexity theory in the occupational therapy literature and they decided to explore the theory further, to see if it would be suitable for their purposes.

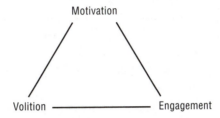

Figure 3.1: Energy source for action cluster

COMPLEXITY THEORY

In order to make sense of the world, people develop theories, such as the theory that the sun orbits around the earth. A theory is 'a conceptual system or framework that is used to organize knowledge and to understand or shape reality' (Creek and Lougher 2008, p.583). Over time, the preferred theory can change as evidence accumulates to suggest that it does not fully explain the situation. An example of this is the shift from people believing the sun moves around the earth to thinking that the earth and the other planets move around the sun.

During the second half of the twentieth century, a new way of thinking began to permeate many disparate disciplines, including meteorology, mathematics, physics and biology (Gleick 1987). This is complexity theory, which:

> offers a way of going beyond the limits of reductionism, because it understands that much of the world is not machine-like and comprehensible through a cataloguing of its parts; but consists instead mostly of organic and holistic systems that are difficult to comprehend by traditional scientific analysis. (Lewin 1993, p.x)

As the new science of complexity gained influence across a wide range of subjects, occupational therapists started to explore its relevance to their own work. For example, a group of occupational scientists proposed that complexity theory would provide an appropriate model for understanding human function and occupation: 'Studies of complex, "dynamic" systems suggest that living systems are self-organizing and pattern forming. Human patterns of occupation may reflect this quality' (Gray, Kennedy and Zemke 1996, p.298).

What is complexity theory?

Several terms have been used to refer to the science of complexity, including chaos theory (Gleick 1987), dynamic systems theory (Gray *et al.* 1996), complexity science (Lewin 1993) and complexity theory (Whiteford, Klomp and Wright-St Clair 2005). The term used throughout this chapter is complexity theory.

The concept of complexity acknowledges that some systems, such as social groups and neural networks, are made up of multiple components that interact both with each other and with the environment. Complex systems 'have the capacity to self-organize their internal structure' (Cilliers 1998, p.25) in response to environmental influences, so that the relationships and interactions between the components of the system shift and change. Such systems, therefore, cannot be fully understood simply by examining the components in isolation: 'Complexity results from the interaction between the components of a system [and] is manifested at the level of the system itself' (Cilliers 1998, pp.2–3).

The European Network of Occupational Therapy in Higher Education (ENOTHE) is an example of a complex system. It is made up of occupational therapists from across Europe who take on a variety of roles within the organization. As the membership of ENOTHE changes over time, so the roles that individual members take also change. It is possible to describe the role of each person within ENOTHE at a particular time but this will not give an understanding of how the whole organization works because what each member does is influenced by what the others do, and this keeps changing. Patterns of interaction and, hence, roles alter over time so that the system evolves in a non-linear way.

A system with a large number of components that interact in a linear fashion is complicated, not complex. An example of a complicated system is a car. It has many components that interact with many other components in complicated ways. However, all these interactions can be expressed and understood as linear equations and the behaviour of the system (the car) is predictable.

Relationships and interactions between components in a complex system are non-linear and unpredictable. An example of a non-linear relationship is the way that a mug of very hot coffee cools to room temperature. The coffee at the top of the mug loses heat to the air and the hotter coffee at the bottom rises to the top, creating a rolling motion in the liquid. There is no linear equation that can predict how quickly the coffee will cool because the speed of cooling affects the rolling motion of the coffee which affects the speed of cooling, and so on. 'Non-linearity means that the act of playing the game has a way of changing the rules' (Gleick 1987, p.24).

Complexity theory and the development of the conceptual framework

Some occupational therapists have represented the relationships between concepts such as *occupation, activity* and *task* as fixed or hierarchical (Hagedorn 2001; Polatajko *et al.* 2004). Through choosing not to work within any one frame of reference or model, terminology group members were free to see that these relationships are not static but are constantly changing, depending on the context and on the perspectives of the observer and of the person engaging in occupational performance. This can be illustrated with an example of the relationship between two terms: *ability* and *skill,* as shown in Example 3.1.

Example 3.1: Dynamic relationship between ability and skill

An *ability* is a personal characteristic that supports occupational performance and a *skill* is an ability developed through practice which enables effective occupational performance. Whether we see something as a skill or an ability shifts and changes as we look at it from different perspectives. Jennifer has an ability to spell, which supports her in editing other people's work, and a skill in technical writing, which has been honed through years of practice and enables her to be a good writer. However, Jennifer's ability to spell has been improved and maintained with practice, so it could be said that her spelling is a skill rather than an ability. Conversely, she is not a particularly good writer when compared with most professional writers who work full time at their writing, so perhaps her writing is more of an ability than a skill.

The realization that the relationships between key occupational therapy concepts are dynamic, not fixed, and that these relationships may be more important than the concepts themselves, led the group to select complexity theory to frame their discussions. Complexity theory provides a way of understanding and articulating the nature of the interactions between concepts so that they can be seen as a whole, complex system: the European conceptual framework for occupational therapy (Figure 3.2).

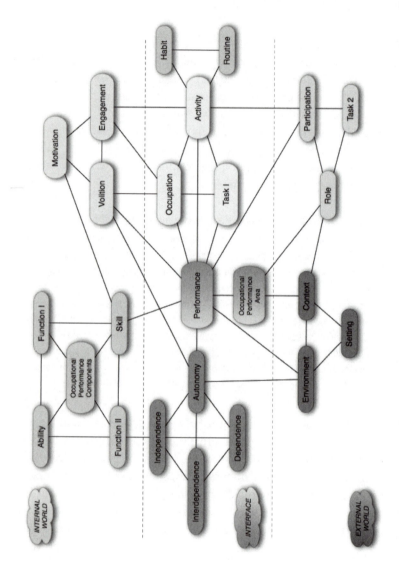

Figure 3.2: The European conceptual framework for occupational therapy

CHARACTERISTICS OF THE EUROPEAN CONCEPTUAL FRAMEWORK FOR OCCUPATIONAL THERAPY

The European conceptual framework is a dynamic, complex system that can be viewed in different ways depending on the context and the person thinking about the framework. It has five characteristics that the reader needs to be aware of in order to understand how it can be used:

1. The meaning of a term can be interpreted from two main perspectives: the observer and performer perspectives.

2. The 25 terms in the framework are clustered into eight groups of closely related concepts.

3. The terms represent aspects of either the performer's internal world or his external world or the interface between these two worlds.

4. The relationships between terms and clusters are dynamic.

5. These relationships change along a series of dimensions.

These five characteristics of the framework will now be described in more detail.

Observer and performer perspectives

During discussions about how the terms relate to each other, group members realized that the way they understood concepts changed depending on whether they were thinking of themselves as performers or as therapists observing someone else's performance (see Example 3.2). This realization highlighted the importance of recognizing which perspective is being taken and that other participants in the situation will have different perspectives.

Example 3.2: Observer and performer perspectives

An occupational therapist could not see the point of studying gardening when she was a student and did not enjoy doing it. There was no meaning and no pleasure for her in gardening and she experienced it as a task that she had to do (performer perspective). Her tutors thought that gardening was an excellent activity through which to teach some of the basic skills and theories of occupational therapy: they saw it as an occupation and were not aware of how the student felt about it (observer perspective).

The European conceptual framework is based on the performer perspective so Chapters 4 to 11, which describe the clusters in the framework, are all written from the performer's perspective. Chapters 12 to 14, in the last section, are written from the therapist's perspective as an observer.

Clusters

The ENOTHE terminology group began their work by isolating key professional concepts and investigating how these were defined in the occupational therapy literature. As the group studied more terms, in more depth, it became apparent that the meanings of individual terms are bounded by the meanings of other, similar terms.

Through the process of comparing and contrasting the precise meanings of concepts, the group eventually composed 25 terms into eight clusters of closely related terms. These are the terms that refer to aspects of the performer's perspective of occupation. Each cluster represents an aspect of the performer's experience, such as the ways that actions are structured and the boundaries to action. Each cluster has been given a descriptive name, as shown in Figure 3.3. For example, the cluster of

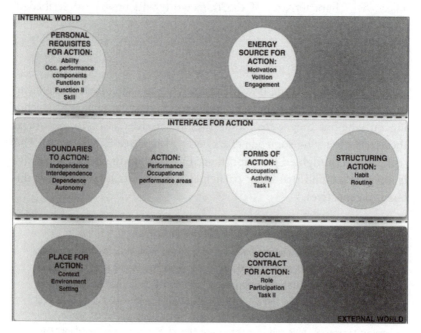

Figure 3.3: The clusters

context, setting and *environment* is called the 'place for action' because all three terms refer to the physical and/or sociocultural surroundings that influence performance (see Box 3.2).

Box 3.2: The place for action cluster

Context, setting and *environment* are all places where action happens but they represent different aspects of place. For example, the concept of *context* can only be fully understood in terms of its similarities to, and differences from, the related concepts of *setting* and *environment*. *Context* refers to the relationships between the environment and other factors that influence the meaning of a task, activity or occupation for the individual. The context of an action determines how the individual interprets what is going on and, hence, how he acts. The *setting* is the immediate surroundings that influence the person's performance. The *environment* is the physical, sociocultural and temporal factors that demand and shape performance. The three terms are closely related but have important differences.

All the terms within a cluster share some of their meanings, in that they relate to a particular aspect of action. For example, *setting, environment* and *context* are all terms that refer to aspects of the physical, social and temporal place for action. Some therapists use closely related terms interchangeably, but an understanding of the precise differences in their meanings allows for clearer thinking and more accurate communication. By having a thorough knowledge of the subtle, or not so subtle, shades of meaning of related terms, the therapist can select the most appropriate one from the cluster to suit the situation.

Each cluster is discussed in detail in its own chapter, in the next section of the book.

Internal and external worlds

Having organized the terms into clusters, the terminology group began to think about how the clusters relate to each other. All action occurs in the 'person-environment interface' (Newman and Holzman 1993, p.24) and the majority of terms refer to this interface, such as *performance, activity* and *autonomy*. However, some terms, such as *motivation* and *function*, refer to the internal world of the performer while others, such as *environment* and *role*, refer to the external world. It is the interaction between the internal and external worlds that leads to action by the individual (Figure 3.4).

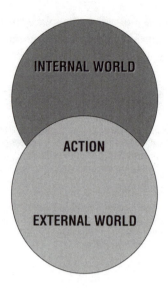

Figure 3.4: Interaction between the internal and external worlds

The internal world of the individual is made up of two clusters of concepts: the individual's emotional energy (energy source for action) and the personal factors that are necessary for performance (personal requisites for action). An example of how an individual's internal world influences performance is given in Example 3.3.

Example 3.3: How the internal world shapes performance

Miguel enjoys physical exercise (*motivation*). His favourite form of exercise is walking but he does not like to walk alone (*volition*), so he has bought a dog to give additional meaning and pleasure to his daily walks (*engagement*). These are his sources of energy for walking.

In order for Miguel to be able to walk every day: he has to be mobile and physically fit (*function 1*); he has to be organized enough to accommodate two walks within his daily routine (*ability*); he has to plan his walks so that they fit into the time available (cognitive *skill*), and he has to control the dog so that it does not get lost or annoy other walkers (psychosocial *skill*). These are some of his personal requisites for the action of walking the dog every day.

The external world of the individual is made up of two clusters: the place where a task, activity or occupation is performed (place for action) and the social supports and constraints on performance (social contract for action). An example of how the external world influences an individual's performance is given in Example 3.4.

Example 3.4: How the external world shapes performance

Miguel lives in the hills so most of his walks are not on flat ground (*environment*). In winter, walking in the snow reminds Miguel of family skiing holidays when he was a child and lifts his spirits (*context*). In summer, the weather is often very hot and humid so that walking is more of a physical effort (*setting*). These are some aspects of the place where his walks are taken.

Not only does Miguel enjoy walking but he also likes meeting other dog owners and has got to know several of them quite well (*participation*). Because Miguel's dog is particularly well behaved, he has gained a reputation for understanding canine behaviour and some of the other owners ask his advice on the best methods of dog training (*role*). Miguel's dog has to be walked every day, and his wife refuses to do it, so Miguel has to go out for a walk even when he does not feel like it (*task 2*). These are some aspects of the social contract for dog walking.

The interface between the internal and external worlds is made up of four clusters: action by the individual (action), the forms that action might take (forms of action), the ways that actions are organized (structuring action) and individual factors that set limits to action (boundaries to action). An example of how an individual's internal world and the external world influence his performance is given in Example 3.5.

Example 3.5: How the interface between internal and external worlds shapes performance

Miguel walks with the dog every day (*performance*) and, for him, it is both a leisure activity and a way of maintaining physical fitness (*occupational performance areas*). These are his actions.

Miguel has freely chosen to keep a dog, knowing that he will have to walk it every day (*autonomy*). He usually finds taking two walks a day well within his capabilities (*independence*). Miguel's neighbour also has a dog and, if one of them is away, they will walk each other's dogs (*interdependence*). For a few days one summer, the police advised people not to walk in the area because it was believed that an escaped convict was hiding there. During that time, Miguel had to use his car and drive to a local park to walk the dog (*dependence* on the car). These are some of the boundaries to him walking the dog every day.

Miguel takes two walks with his dog each day, in the morning and again in the evening (*activity*). On most days, he feels that taking two long walks a day is an appropriate activity for a fit, active person like himself: it is enjoyable, it keeps the dog healthy and it provides opportunities for him to talk with other dog owners (*occupation*). However, on some days he has other, more important things to do so he perceives walking the dog as an unwelcome imposition (*task 2*). Activities, occupations and tasks are different forms of action in the performer's mind, even though the performance may look the same.

Miguel has breakfast when he first gets up in the morning, then takes the dog for a walk before he goes to work (*routine*). Because he only has half an hour for the morning walk, he takes the same route every day without thinking about it (*habit*). In the evenings, after work, he has time to try different paths and vary the length of his walks. These are some of the ways in which Miguel structures the action of walking the dog.

Dynamic relationships between terms

Relationships between terms in the European conceptual framework for occupational therapy are not static but will change depending on the context in which the framework is being used. Two examples of this are given here: forming new clusters and concepts moving between worlds.

Within the conceptual framework, all the terms relate to all the other terms, although some of them are closer in meaning than others. Concepts that are closer in meaning to each other are clustered together. However, changing circumstances can weaken or strengthen the relationships between different concepts so that new clusters are formed, as described in Example 3.6.

Example 3.6: Relationships between concepts

Miguel's skill in handling dogs has given him a high status role among the local dog owners that enhances his sense both of engagement in the activity of dog walking and of participation in the local community. For Miguel, dog walking creates strong relationships between the concepts of *skill, role, engagement* and *participation* so that these concepts, in the context of his daily walks, form a new cluster.

Terms that are located within the interface between the internal and external worlds in the framework can be conceptualized as belonging, in certain instances, to another world or may even be in more than one world at the same time, as illustrated in Example 3.7.

Example 3.7: Movement between worlds

Autonomy is the freedom to make choices based on consideration of internal and external circumstances and to act on those choices. Miguel freely chose to buy a dog, knowing that he would have to walk it twice a day: his choice was autonomous. That autonomy was based not only on consideration of his need for exercise and his desire for company on his walks (internal circumstances) but also on knowledge and consideration of his wife's views on dogs, the suitability of their house for a dog and the nearness of appropriate spaces for dog walking (external circumstances). When making his choice, the overriding consideration for Miguel was how his wife felt about them keeping a dog, which shifted the concept of autonomy, for this particular issue, closer to the external world than the internal world.

Dimensions

The concept of dimensions is used to explain the relationships between terms within a cluster. Dimensions are the attributes of terms that clarify the differences between them: through understanding the dimensions along which the terms within a cluster interact, we can see more clearly the precise differences between them. For example, some of the difference between *occupation* and *occupational performance* can be understood from their relative positions on the abstract–concrete continuum. Occupational performance is what the person is doing, such as cooking a meal (more concrete). Occupation is how the person conceptualizes what she or he is doing, such as experiencing cooking as a task to be accomplished or as an occupation to be relished (more abstract). It is possible to identify a number of dimensions along which the terms relate to each other, as shown in Figure 3.5.

Abstract–Concrete

Meaning–No meaning

Observable–Non-observable

Physical environment–Sociocultural environment

Spatiotemporal–Not spatiotemporal

Whole–Part

Complex–Simple

Figure 3.5: Dimensions that influence relationships within the framework

Most of these dimensions represent a continuum rather than a binary opposition. An example is the continuum of meaning–no meaning: we can talk about degrees of meaning, as shown in Example 3.8. The observable–non-observable dimension represents opposites: for example, occupational performance is observable but occupation is the idea of a group of activities that has personal and sociocultural meaning and is not observable.

Example 3.8: Continuum of meaning–no meaning

Miguel enjoys physical exercise but finds that the activity of walking his dog has more personal meaning than the activity of going to the gym. The degree and type of meaning that a particular activity holds might be different on different occasions, depending on Miguel's intentions and on the context. For example, when Miguel has been working on the computer all day, he experiences his evening walk as liberation from hard labour. However, at the weekend, when he has been gardening all day and is tired, the physical exertion of walking the dog feels more like a punishment.

Another dimension, which is linked to the abstract–concrete and observable–non-observable dimensions, is the physical environment–socio-cultural environment dimension. For example, occupations exist in a sociocultural environment while task performance takes place in a physical environment, as described in Example 3.9.

Example 3.9: Continuum of physical environment–sociocultural environment

Owning a dog is an occupation for Miguel, and occupational performance takes place within social and cultural environments. For example, Miguel has earned a reputation for being good with dogs because he and his dog went together to a training school for several months and learned the most up-to-date and evidence-based methods of dog handling.

Putting a lead on the dog so that he can take it for a walk is a task that Miguel performs. Task performance takes place in a physical environment, such as when Miguel puts a lead on his dog to keep it safe if they walk near a road.

Some of the terms in the conceptual framework have a spatiotemporal dimension while others are not spatiotemporal. See Example 3.10.

Example 3.10: Continuum of spatiotemporal–not spatiotemporal

In order to take different routes for his daily walks, Miguel needs various cognitive functions such as planning, sequencing, timing and visualizing: these functions are potentials, which are available all the time even when he is not using them. Function does not have a temporal dimension; it can be specific to certain times but it does not have duration. Walking, on the other hand, is an activity, which has a temporal dimension in that it takes place over time. The length of time for the walk can vary, being shorter when Miguel is in a hurry to get to work or longer at the weekend when he is enjoying the activity.

If we explore terms along the dimension of whole–part, we see that everything is both a part and a whole. Whether something is seen as a part or a whole depends on the perceptions of the person performing the activity, as illustrated in Example 3.11.

Example 3.11: Continuum of whole–part

Walking the dog is a whole activity made up of a sequence of tasks, which include: putting on outdoor clothing, finding the lead, putting it on the dog, leaving the house, walking, returning to the house and cleaning muddy footwear.

Walking the dog is also a part of the occupation of dog owner, which involves other activities such as shopping for dog food, finding a suitable kennel for holiday care, brushing the dog and taking it to the vet.

The final dimension to consider is complex–simple. For example, choosing what task to do is a relatively simple process, with the choice being shaped by the physical environment, the activity and the immediate goal. Choosing occupations requires a more complex interaction between many factors. The immediate goals of an occupation usually have longer–term goals behind them; concrete goals can represent more symbolic goals, and the participants in a situation may all have very different goals, as described in Example 3.12.

Example 3.12: Continuum of complex–simple

For Miguel, taking on the occupation of owning a dog was the outcome of many complex deliberations. He and his wife chose to live in a village, in part so that Miguel would be able to go walking regularly. He considered joining a walking group, rather than buying a dog, but most groups only go walking once a week. He tried to persuade his wife to walk with him but she prefers going to the gym. When he first had the idea of getting a dog, Miguel thought about what breed to buy, whether the dog could be left at home while he was at work, where it could stay while the couple were away on holiday and other practical considerations.

In contrast, Miguel sees cleaning up after his dog as a task, and choosing what task to do is a relatively simple process. When the dog defecates on or near the path, Miguel clears up the mess using a plastic bag which he then puts into the next dog bin. When the dog defecates in the undergrowth, Miguel does not attempt to clear up the mess.

Six dimensions have been described here that can be used to deepen our understanding of occupational therapy concepts when reflecting on the meanings of terms and exploring their characteristics.

SUMMARY

This chapter began with a brief account of the method used by the terminology working group to select key occupational therapy terms, construct consensus definitions in English and translate the definitions into other European languages. The definitions were listed but the reader is advised that a more detailed account of the meaning of the different terms can be found in Chapters 4 to 11.

The next section of the chapter gave an outline of complexity theory, showing how it was used to inform the development of the European conceptual framework. The framework was presented and its key characteristics were explained: observer and performer perspectives; clusters; internal and external worlds; relationships between the terms, and dimensions. In order to use the framework to inform practice, it is necessary to understand these five characteristics, which together account for the fluid, provisional nature of the framework.

Each of the next eight chapters explores in depth one of the eight clusters of terms in the conceptual framework.

REFERENCES

Cilliers, P. (1998) *Complexity and Postmodernism: Understanding Complex Systems.* London: Routledge.

Creek, J. and Lougher, L. (eds) (2008) *Occupational Therapy and Mental Health, Fourth Edition.* Edinburgh: Churchill Livingstone Elsevier.

de Witt, P. (2005) 'Creative ability: a model for psychosocial occupational therapy.' In R. Crouch and V. Alers (eds) *Occupational Therapy in Psychiatry and Mental Health, Fourth Edition.* London: Whurr.

Dickoff, J. and James, P. (1968) 'A theory of theories: a position paper.' *Nursing Research 17,* 3, 197–203.

Dickoff, J., James, P. and Wiedenbach, E. (1968) 'Theory in a practice discipline: Part 1. Practice oriented theory.' *Nursing Research 17,* 5, 415–435.

du Toit, V. (1991) *Patient Volition and Action in Occupational Therapy.* Hillbrow, SA: Vona & Marie du Toit Foundation.

Gleick, J. (1987) *Chaos: Making a New Science.* London: Abacus.

Gray, J.M., Kennedy, B.L. and Zemke, R. (1996) 'Dynamic systems theory: an overview.' In R. Zemke and F. Clark (eds) *Occupational Science: The Evolving Discipline.* Philadelphia, PA: F.A. Davis.

Hagedorn, R. (2001) *Foundations for Practice in Occupational Therapy, Third Edition.* Edinburgh: Churchill Livingstone.

Lewin, R. (1993) *Complexity: Life at the Edge of Chaos, Second Edition.* Guernsey: Phoenix.

Newman, F. and Holzman, L. (1993) *Lev Vygotsky: Revolutionary Scientist.* London: Routledge.

Polatajko, H.J., Davis, J.A., Hobson, S.J.G., Landry, J.E, *et al.* (2004) 'Meeting the responsibility that comes with the privilege: introducing a taxonomic code for understanding occupation.' *Canadian Journal of Occupational Therapy 71,* 5, 261–264.

Whiteford, G., Klomp, N. and Wright-St Clair, V. (2005) 'Complexity theory: understanding occupation, practice and context.' In G. Whiteford and V. Wright-St Clair (eds) *Occupation and Practice in Context.* Sydney: Elsevier Churchill Livingstone.

SECTION 2

THE PERFORMER'S PERSPECTIVE

This section of the book describes the European conceptual framework in detail. As explained in Chapter 3, the framework is made up of eight clusters of terms, each of which refers to an aspect of occupation. The chapters in this section explore the meaning of the terms and explain the relationships between them.

The European conceptual framework presents an explanation of occupation from the perspective of the performer, not that of the observer. The way that terms and concepts are understood will change when we shift from thinking about ourselves performing an occupation to observing someone else's performance. The perspective of the therapist, as observer, is described in Section 3 of the book.

The chapters in this section all have the same structure. For each term in the cluster, the common usage of the term is discussed, followed by an exploration of the way that it is used by occupational therapists. The European definition of the term is then given, with an explanation of how it was developed. The last part of the chapter examines the relationships between the terms in the cluster, looking at what they have in common and how their meanings differ. Examples are given of how these relationships shift and change depending on the context in which actions are performed and on the perspective of the performer.

The chapters in Section 2 do not have to be read in any particular order. Each chapter describes one cluster of terms in detail, and they all stand alone. Chapters 4 to 7 describe the four clusters of terms in the interface between the internal and external worlds of the performer. Chapters 8 and 9 describe the two clusters of terms in the internal world of the performer. Chapters 10 and 11 describe the two clusters of terms in the external world of the performer.

CHAPTER 4

FORMS OF ACTION

INTRODUCTION

The purpose of this chapter, together with the next three chapters, is to explore the interface between the internal and external worlds of the performer where action, or doing, takes place. This is the largest section of the conceptual framework: it represents the active dimension of human beings through which they 'develop skills, exercise and test their capacities, interact with others, adapt to circumstances, meet basic vital needs, express who they are and strive towards reaching their goals' (College of Occupational Therapists 2006, p.3).

Occupational therapists position themselves as experts in doing. Therefore the profession must have a specialized vocabulary of words that refer to different aspects of doing. We need to define these words clearly and to differentiate between them.

In common usage, human activity is described in words such as movement, action, participation, play, work, education and leisure. Occupational therapists have their own terms: occupation, activity, task, performance, performance areas, habit and routine. None of these terms has been coined by occupational therapists, although they are used in a specialist sense within the profession, and the professional meanings of the terms are not widely understood outside occupational therapy.

Within occupational therapy, there is no agreement about the precise meanings of the words we use to describe our core purpose and practice. Definitions of occupation and activity abound in the literature, making it impossible to agree on how different aspects of doing relate to each other. The most common conceptualization is that occupation, activity and task exist in a fixed hierarchical relationship (Golledge 1998; Hagedorn 2000; Polatajko *et al.* 2004), but no static framework can suit all purposes because human action is always based on, and influenced by, numerous factors that interact in complex ways.

For occupational therapists to be able to communicate among ourselves, and with others, about occupation as an essential part of human life, we need a vocabulary that captures the complexity of the concept. The words that we use must allow us to think clearly about the nature of human doing and to express shades of meaning accurately.

This chapter explores both the common and the specialized meanings of three terms: *occupation, activity* and *task*. These are the words that are used by occupational therapists to refer to forms of action.

OCCUPATION

The word *occupation* was chosen by the founders of the profession to represent the core concept underpinning our practice and the main focus of our interventions. Occupational therapists have worked hard to reach a full understanding of this word and to define it in a way that captures the centrality of occupation to human development and experience. Most importantly, we have struggled to achieve a wider understanding of our professional meanings among other health care professionals and the general public. These issues are discussed in this section.

What occupation means in common usage

According to the *New Shorter Oxford English Dictionary* (1993), the word *occupation* has four distinct meanings:

1. The state of having one's time or attention occupied; employment. What a person is (habitually) engaged in, esp. to earn a living; a job; a business; a profession; a pursuit; an activity.

2. The action or condition of residing in or holding a place or position; the state of being so occupied; tenure, occupancy.

3. Use, employment (of a thing).

4. The action of taking or maintaining possession of a country, building, etc., by force; the state of being so occupied; the duration or an instance of this.

Most people think of work or employment when they hear the word *occupation*. This is the meaning that is most often assumed by the general public when occupational therapy is mentioned: it is thought to be a profession that is concerned with people's ability to work, like occupational health. The second meaning, tenure or occupancy, is frequently used when referring to someone holding a physical space; for example, we talk about the occupation of a public building as a form of protest or about signs of occupation in a house.

Occupation is not commonly used in its third sense and the *New Shorter Oxford English Dictionary* (1993) does not give any examples of this usage. The fourth meaning is commonly used to refer to the invading force that stays in a country, as in the occupation of Palestinian territories by Israel. This meaning is so widely recognized that there may be reluctance to use the word *occupation* in any other sense in countries that have experienced this condition. An occupational therapist, Barbara Lavin (2005), played on the first and fourth meanings of the term when she wrote a paper called: 'Occupation under occupation: days of conflict and curfew in Bethlehem.'

In the minds of most people in the UK, including health and social care staff, occupation means employment. Other types of occupation are referred to individually, for example education, leisure or activities of daily living. The people who use occupational therapy services are more likely to refer to the things they do every day as activities. The terms used in health and social care settings that perhaps come closest to the meaning of occupation, as it is understood by occupational therapists, are participation and lifestyle. These words have been appearing more frequently, in recent years, in policy documents and research papers, especially when describing research into health promotion. For example, a report on mental health and social exclusion (Social Exclusion Unit 2004, p.83) referred to 'participation in arts' and the report of a review of public health in England (Wanless 2004, p.6) identified 'lifestyle determinants of future health'.

How occupational therapists use the term occupation

The way that occupational therapists understand the concept of occupation is influenced by their own language and culture, so it is not always possible to translate the word directly and retain the meaning that it has in English. For example, Iwama (2006, p.23) suggested that, to a Japanese person, occupation means 'work of the tedious and laborious kind'.

Many definitions of occupation can be found in the occupational therapy literature. For example, ten definitions, taken from different sources, were cited in the UK occupational therapy standard terminology project report (College of Occupational Therapists 2004). This project identified the most common elements from all these definitions and used them to produce an eleventh one: 'an occupation is an activity or group of activities that engages a person in everyday life, has personal meaning and provides structure to time' (*ibid.*, p.2).

Although every occupational therapy author seems to produce a new definition of occupation, there is an increasing use of the same words and phrases in all of them, suggesting a convergence of opinion on the meaning of occupation. Some of these words and phrases are shown in Box 4.1.

Box 4.1: Words and phrases used in definitions of occupation

Daily activities	Structure
Tasks	Organization of time and effort
Everyday life	Goal directed
Persons of any age	Meets needs
Personal meaning	Allows adaptation
Sociocultural meaning	Defines a sphere of action
Individual value	Extends over time
Cultural values	Personal care
Part of personal identity	Productivity
Part of social identity	Leisure

The occupational therapy theorist Hagedorn (2000) described a taxonomy of occupation consisting of three levels, in which the lower levels are incorporated into the higher ones, as shown in Figure 4.1. The highest rank, the organizational level, is made up of social roles, 'which direct the individual's engagement in certain activities or tasks related to the role over extended periods of time' (p.26), and occupations, which are 'a form of human endeavour which provides longitudinal organization of time and effort in a person's life' (p.309). These definitions do not make a clear difference between a role and an occupation.

Level of occupation	Organizing structure
Organizational	Social roles
	Occupations
Effective	Routines
	Activities
Developmental	
	Tasks
Constructive	Task stages
Acquisitional	Performance unit
	Actions
Proto-occupational	Interactions
	Reactions
	Skill components

Figure 4.1: Levels of occupation (adapted from Hagedorn 2000)

The UK project to define occupational therapy as a complex intervention (Creek 2003) represents a change in the way that occupational therapists think about occupation. The project report describes occupation as 'complex and multifaceted, incorporating physical, social, psychological, emotional and spiritual dimensions' (p.32). These dimensions do not exist in a hierarchical relationship but interact with each other in complex ways so that 'the initiation, expression and carrying out of occupation is...mostly unique to the individual' (p.33).

Alongside developing an interest in the complexity of occupation, occupational therapists have also embraced the *International Classification of Functioning, Disability and Health* (World Health Organization 2001) and begun to incorporate its framework and terminology into descriptions of their own practice (McDonald, Surtees and Wirz 2004). For example, occupational therapists now talk about people participating in life situations through their occupations. Further discussion of the concept of *participation* can be found in Chapter 10.

How occupation is understood within the conceptual framework

The European definition of *occupation* was constructed from existing definitions of the term:

. . . .

An *occupation* is a group of activities that has personal and sociocultural meaning, is named within a culture and supports participation in society. Occupations can be categorized as self-care, productivity and/or leisure.

. . . .

This definition contains six elements:

- a group of activities
- has personal meaning
- has sociocultural meaning
- is named within a culture
- supports participation in society
- can be categorized as self-care, productivity and/or leisure.

An occupation is not a performance and therefore, while occupations can be described or discussed, they cannot be observed. Occupations are ideas or concepts that can be enacted through the activities that are their doing aspects; it is the performance of activities that we observe. For example, Johanna has many occupations, one of which is housekeeping. Some of the activities that Johanna performs as part of this occupation include: tidying, cleaning, cooking, washing up, gardening, decorating, household shopping and organizing house maintenance.

The activities that a person performs in support of an occupation exist in a dynamic relationship that changes over time through the influence of personal and cultural characteristics. For example, the way that people listen to music often changes as they get older, and societies change over time so that the personal sound systems used today bear little relationship to the transistor radio of 40 years ago.

An occupation has meaning for the person who engages in it. Meaning is the significance or importance that the occupation has for the individual (*New Shorter Oxford English Dictionary* 1993), which may be personal or sociocultural or both. For example, the personal meaning of making a cup of tea might be to:

- express hospitality to a visitor
- satisfy personal preferences by brewing one's favourite kind of tea

- be the same kind of housewife as one's mother

- take a break from work

- all of these.

Making a cup of tea also has layers of sociocultural meaning that are linked to the purpose, materials, tools, methods and context. These might include the reason for making the tea, the type of tea used, the implements used, the method of making it, the time of day it is drunk, the location, the company and so on.

Personal and cultural meanings are closely linked to each other and together influence the occupations that people choose to engage in. A person might take up an occupation because it enhances his sense of identity and self-esteem; or because it is expected of him at this time and place in his life; or because the occupation will help him to participate more fully in his social group, or for all these reasons (Figure 4.2). For example, Sylvie might join a slimming club because she would like to be thinner, because her doctor says that she must lose weight for the sake of her health, or because her best friends all attend one regularly.

Different intensity of meaning may be attached to different occupations and to the same occupation at different times, depending on the context. For example, Joaquim loves most sports but attending a football match has more meaning for him than watching tennis. Football has both personal and sociocultural meanings for Joaquim, and those meanings are especially powerful when he is watching his home team play.

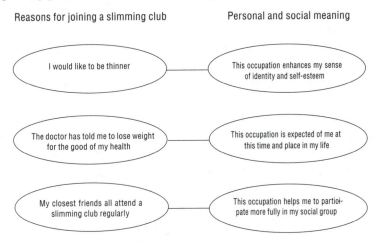

Reasons for joining a slimming club   Personal and social meaning

I would like to be thinner

This occupation enhances my sense of identity and self-esteem

The doctor has told me to lose weight for the good of my health

This occupation is expected of me at this time and place in my life

My closest friends all attend a slimming club regularly

This occupation helps me to participate more fully in my social group

Figure 4.2: Meanings influencing why someone takes up an occupation

Occupations exist and have meaning within a culture, even if only some of the population perform them. For example, driving exists and has both personal and sociocultural meanings for people who do not drive, such as children. Each person needs to understand the social and cultural meanings of the most common or most valued occupations performed within his culture in order to be a part of it. For example, when a major international sporting event, like the Olympic Games or the football world cup, is held in a country, everyone becomes involved to some extent, not just those who are normally interested in sport.

Understanding the meaning of an occupation for others, even if a person does not engage in it himself, can be a way of participating in society. Peter does not have a garden but he appreciates the importance of gardening to his friends and is happy to talk about it with them.

Engagement in an occupation does not have to include the direct performance of activities. It is possible to be involved peripherally by being the commentator rather than the sportsman, making tea at a cricket match rather than playing the game, or just watching the match on television. People choose whether or not to engage in occupations, and how they will participate, for various reasons. The meanings ascribed to a particular occupation can be positive, leading people to participate in it, or negative, leading them away from participation. The meanings given to occupations may be related to culture, gender, age and personal or social influences. For example, a man may view certain occupations as being women's work within his culture and refuse to do them because he does not want to be seen as effeminate. Finding positive meaning in a range of socially and culturally valued occupations supports participation in society.

Occupations are named within a culture and these names are often verbs, such as gardening, cooking, parenting and horse racing. Some occupations, such as looking after children and preparing food, are found in all cultures, so that we might expect to find a name for them in all languages. Other occupations, such as tending a loom in a cotton mill or leading a camel caravan, are specific to certain cultures and may not have a name in other languages. Occupations can disappear as society changes, so that the names become obsolete. An example of this is fulling, which means thickening cloth by beating it. This function is now performed by machinery so that we no longer have fullers – people with the occupation of fulling – in the United Kingdom.

Occupations support the individual's participation in the life of his community by providing a recognized framework for performing the socially and culturally acceptable activities that embed the person in his social context. For example, doing occupational therapy enables Jennifer to earn a living, it contributes to her social status and it is an important vehicle through which she can make social, economic and productive contributions to her community.

Occupations can be categorized as self-care, productivity and/or leisure, but a single occupation may be located in more than one category, even for the same person. For example, dressmaking can be a hobby (leisure), it can contribute to grooming (self-care) and it can be done for other people in order to earn money (productivity). Even for an individual, the categories are fluid and an occupation can fit better in one or another depending on the context.

This section has illustrated the complex and dynamic nature of occupation through examining what the term means in common usage, the ways that occupational therapists use it and how the concept fits into the European conceptual framework. The next section examines the concept of *activity*.

ACTIVITY

The way that occupational therapists use the word *activity* is much closer in meaning to common usage than their understanding of the word *occupation*. This section will discuss the different ways in which the term is used by the general public, by occupational therapists and within this conceptual framework.

What activity means in common usage

The word *activity* has four meanings, according to the *New Shorter Oxford English Dictionary* (1993):

1. The state of being active; the exertion of energy, action.

2. Brisk or vigorous action; energy; diligence; liveliness.

3. Gymnastics, athletics; a gymnastic exercise.

4. An active force or operation; an occupation, a pursuit.

It can be seen from these definitions that activity is understood to mean physical exertion, usually vigorous in nature. This is often the way that the term is used by the general public, and the word exercise may be used synonymously with physical activity.

However, policy documents that are concerned with the impact of activity on health usually specify if they are referring to physical activity or to other types of activity. For example, a report from the Chief Medical Officer (Department of Health 2004) is subtitled 'Evidence on the impact of physical activity and its relationship to health'. A research paper describing a study of people with Alzheimer's disease classified activities into 'intellectual, passive, and physical' categories (Friedland *et al.* 2001, p.3440).

Other words that are used to refer to activity include pursuit, as in 'creative pursuits' (Department of Health 2004, p.175), and endeavour, as in 'leisure endeavors [sic]' (Friedland *et al.* 2001, p.3440).

Intensive public health programmes to educate people about the importance of healthy lifestyles appear to have connected activity, in the sense of exercise, with health in the minds of the public. For example, advice given in a magazine for keeping healthy in the winter includes: 'people who exercise regularly [are] less prone to depression. And that doesn't have to be major athletics or aerobic acrobatics, but just walking or other gentle activities' (Cullen 2005, p.9).

The *International Classification of Functioning, Disability and Health* (ICF) (World Health Organization 2001, p.10) defines activity in a narrower sense as: 'the execution of a task or action by an individual'. The use of the term *activity* as one of the main components of the ICF has been significant for occupational therapists in that it has drawn attention to the importance of activity for health.

How occupational therapists use the term activity

In the 1990s, at a time when occupational therapists began to reject the use of the word activity to describe our main tool for intervention but were not yet comfortable with talking about occupation, the phrase 'purposeful activity' came into vogue (Creek 1998; Golledge 1998). Creek (1998, p.17) defined purposeful activity as 'actions that are directed towards a goal or end result'.

The word purposeful is mainly redundant, since it is difficult to think of an activity that does not have a purpose. Nevertheless, the phrase purposeful activity is still seen in the occupational therapy literature, sometimes used interchangeably with activity (Smith 2005; Wenborn 2005) or with occupation (Long 2004). This may be because occupational therapists confuse purpose and meaning. The purpose of an activity is its goal and is a part of the activity (Creek 2008). For example, the purpose of cooking a meal is to produce dinner for the family. The meaning of an activity is its significance or importance (Creek 2003) and this is located in the person doing the activity. The meaning of an activity may, therefore, be different for different people and for the same person on different occasions. For example, watching a game of football represents excitement, shared social values and national pride for Joaquim, while to Jennifer it is usually boring and irrelevant to her life. However, when Jennifer visited Portugal for the first time, her hosts took her to dinner in a restaurant where they could watch their national team play in the European cup, and she enjoyed watching the match as part of the whole experience.

Those occupational therapists who use both the terms *occupation* and *activity* often define them by their similarities and differences to each other. For example, Long (2004) suggested that a key difference between occupation and activity is that occupations always have meaning and purpose while activities can lack both.

For many years, occupational therapy theorists have described different types of performance existing in a fixed hierarchical relationship, with the higher levels incorporating the lower levels. For example, Golledge (1998) put occupation at the highest level followed by purposeful activity, activity and, at the lowest level, diversional activity. Hagedorn (2000) proposed a taxonomy of occupation in which activities are ranked between occupations and tasks (Figure 4.1).

Two Danish occupational therapists, Fortmeier and Thanning (2002), offered a different understanding of activity, based on the activity theory developed by Russian psychologists such as Leont'ev and Vygotsky. In this theory, activity is described as the medium through which each individual interacts with the world:

> Every human being develops throughout his life via his *activity*... Through his actions, the person also changes his environment, at the same time developing and changing his own action possibilities. (Fortmeier and Thanning 2002, pp.27–28)

This specialized conceptualization of activity has much to offer occupational therapists in explaining why doing is crucial for health and well-being. However, it is different from the way that occupational therapists have traditionally understood the term and from how it is defined within the European conceptual framework.

How activity is understood within the conceptual framework

The European definition of *activity* was constructed from existing definitions of the term. This section presents the definition, describes how it was developed and explores its meaning, using examples from life.

· ·

An *activity* is a structured series of actions or tasks that contribute to occupations.

· ·

This definition was constructed from three elements that were found in existing definitions of activity:

- contribute to occupations

- structured

- a series of actions or tasks.

Activities do not contribute to occupations in the sense of being lesser parts of them. It is not possible to understand an occupation by analysing it into its component activities because these activities will vary from person to person and in the same person over time. For example, when Jennifer first became an occupational therapist, most of the activities she performed as part of this occupation involved direct patient contact, communication with colleagues or record keeping. Although she still has the same occupation, her activities today are very different, being mainly to do with research, teaching and writing.

A single activity may contribute to more than one occupation, sequentially or simultaneously. Hilde can make a cup of tea to have with breakfast so that it contributes to her self-care, or she can make a cup of tea with a client so that it is part of her main work occupation: occupational therapy. When the client comes for a breakfast meeting with Hilde, making a cup of tea contributes to both self-care and work occupations at the same time.

An activity is a doing process that is structured towards a goal; it is not a random series of actions. For example, the activity of making a cup of tea consists of a series of tasks – filling the kettle and switching it on, putting tea leaves in the pot, setting out the cup and saucer, putting milk in a jug and so on – that are performed in a sequence leading to the goal being achieved. If the tasks are not performed in the right sequence, or if one or more tasks are missed out, the activity will not be completed successfully. However, the same activity may be structured in many different ways depending on personal preferences, the constraints of the physical environment or social custom. Making a cup of tea is the same activity in England, Spain, India or Japan but the tools, the tasks and the sequence of tasks may vary.

The sequence of tasks in an activity tends to be the same each time an individual performs it, because people develop routines. However, this sequence is not fixed and can be adapted to changing circumstances and meanings. Routines allow us to carry out our daily activities efficiently but they can be a problem if they are too rigid, as we become unable to adapt to circumstances. Further discussion of the concept of *routine* can be found in Chapter 6.

The definition of activity does not include meaning because activities are performed in order to contribute to occupations. Therefore the meaning of an activity comes from the occupation to which it is contributing. Since an activity can contribute to many different occupations, and to more than one occupation at the same time, the meaning of an activity may be different each time it is performed.

TASK

When the terminology group began to analyse existing definitions of *task*, they discovered that occupational therapists use it in two distinct ways: one is closely related to *occupation* and *activity* in the cluster of doing terms; the other is nearer in meaning to the dictionary definition of the term. This section presents the first definition of *task*, describes how it was developed and explores its meaning, using examples from life. The second definition is discussed in Chapter 10.

What task means in common usage

In common usage, a task is 'a piece of work imposed on or undertaken by a person; a fixed quantity of labour to be performed by a person' (*New Shorter Oxford English Dictionary* 1993). This definition indicates that although a person can freely undertake a task it is often perceived as an imposition, as when the teacher sets a homework task for the class. The word may also carry an implication of being difficult to do, for example, when someone takes on the task of turning around a failing business. This meaning of the word *task* is explored further in Chapter 10.

The ICF (World Health Organization 2001, p.10) includes a *task* in its definition of *activity*: 'Activity is the execution of a task or action by an individual'.

How occupational therapists use the term task

For occupational therapists, the concept of task seems to be less problematic than many other words within the conceptual framework. In the occupational therapy literature, it is commonly used to describe a component or stage of an activity, for example, 'Daily life consists of engaging in **tasks** to perform **activities** required by occupations' (Harvey and Pentland 2004, p.64). When the word is used in this way, it is defined as: 'A constituent part of an activity' (Creek 2002, p.588) or 'A self-contained stage in an activity, or a self-contained piece of performance with a completed purpose or product' (Hagedorn 2000, p.311).

Both these writers define a task as part of an activity. However, as explained in the last section, Hagedorn's taxonomy of occupation is a hierarchical one in which task has a lower ranking than activity (Figure 4.1). This is different from the way that the relationships between occupations, activities and tasks are conceptualized in the European framework.

Some writers have used the word skill in a similar sense to the way that Hagedorn and Creek use task (Forsyth and Kielhofner 2006). The meaning of *skill* is explored in more depth in Chapter 8.

How task is understood within the conceptual framework

. . . .

A *task* is a series of structured steps (actions and/or thoughts) intended to accomplish the performance of an activity.

. . . .

This definition was constructed from four elements that were found in existing definitions of task:

- a series of structured steps

- actions and/or thoughts

- intentional

- to accomplish the performance of an activity.

A task is performed in a structured series of steps towards a particular goal. For example, the first task in making a cup of tea may be to fill the kettle. This involves checking the water level, picking up the kettle, taking it to the sink, holding it under the tap, turning on the tap and so on. If these steps are not performed in the correct sequence, or if one or more steps are missed out, the task of filling the kettle will not be completed successfully.

A task is made up of steps which may be actions, thoughts or a mixture of both. For example, one step in making a cup of tea may be to make a decision about which type of tea to have. Filling the kettle and choosing the type of tea are both steps but the first is a physical action and the second is a thought process.

The person carrying out a task has intentions. To intend means to have a purpose, therefore tasks are intentional because they are voluntary and are carried out for a purpose. Each task has its own purpose, such as filling the kettle, but also shares the overall purpose of accomplishing the performance of an activity, in this case making a cup of tea.

To accomplish something means to complete it. Carrying out a single task in isolation will not lead to the accomplishment of an activity without the other tasks in the series. For example, filling the kettle by itself will not produce a cup of tea. Equally, carrying out a single step in a task, such as picking up the kettle, will not accomplish the task without completing the necessary series of steps. Repetition of single steps or tasks that do not lead to the accomplishment of an activity is called stereotypical behaviour and may be caused by a disorder such as epilepsy, schizophrenia or autism.

This section has explored the meaning of the word *task*, as it is defined in the *New Shorter Oxford English Dictionary* and used by the general population. It has demonstrated that occupational therapists use the term in two different ways and has explored the European definition of the first meaning of task. The next section looks at the relationships between the three terms that represent forms of action.

RELATIONSHIPS BETWEEN THE TERMS REPRESENTING FORMS OF ACTION

Occupational therapists need a specialized vocabulary for referring to forms of action, or doing, in order to be able to build theories that are adequate for the purposes of practice, education and research. In this chapter, we have seen how, for many years, occupational therapists have conceptualized occupations, activities and tasks as relating to each other in a hierarchical taxonomy, in which each higher term incorporates those at the lower levels (Creek 2002; Golledge 1998; Polatajko *et al.* 2004). For example, Hagedorn (2000) outlined a taxonomy of 11 terms that represent levels of occupational performance, with social roles at the highest level and skill components at the lowest level (Figure 4.1). In this classification, a social role organizes the lower levels of performance by 'direct[ing] the individual's engagement in certain occupations, activities or tasks related to the role' (Hagedorn 2000, p.26).

As described in Chapter 3, the European conceptual framework for occupational therapy takes a different view of how occupations, activities and tasks relate to each other. The framework conceptualizes these relationships as constantly changing, depending on the perspective taken by the performer and on the context of the performance. What people do and how they do it are influenced by a multitude of internal and external factors, as described in Chapters 8 to 11. A change in one factor can have an unpredictable impact on all the other factors, as well as having a direct effect on performance, as shown in Example 4.1. This means that the different forms of action relate to each other in complex, dynamic ways.

Example 4.1: How Mrs Smith regained her independence

Mrs Smith lived alone, after the death of her husband, in a two-bedroom terraced house in a small town. She was independent in self-care, household management and using public transport.

Following an episode of diarrhoea and vomiting, Mrs Smith became paralysed from the neck down and was diagnosed with Guillain-Barré syndrome. She survived the acute phase but was not able to walk without a frame, to manage stairs or to do her own shopping. The occupational therapist did a home visit with Mrs Smith and made the judgement that it would not be safe for her to be discharged to her home.

Mrs Smith was very reluctant to give up her house. She agreed to a period of convalescence in a small, local hospital where she became depressed and bed bound. However, her friends were able to visit every day and they made a plan to assist Mrs Smith with her housework and shopping. With the renewed possibility of going home, Mrs Smith became keen to explore alternative ways of getting up and down stairs. The occupational therapist carried out another home visit with her and recommended some minor adaptations to the house to make it more accessible. Mrs Smith was eventually discharged home with some social support.

The move from a city hospital to one in Mrs Smith's own town made it possible for her friends to visit regularly and see what problems she faced. Their positive intervention gave Mrs Smith the incentive to work hard at her rehabilitation.

Mrs Smith's physical improvement then persuaded the occupational therapist to reconsider the viability of her returning to live in her own home.

Some occupational therapists use the three terms representing forms of action interchangeably, but there is practical value in differentiating between them. The occupational therapist has to try to elicit the meaning that an action, or set of actions, has for the client, so that we understand whether he experiences it as an occupation, an activity or a task. We may choose to work with both our own understanding of the client's performance and with his understanding of it, but it is important to be clear about whose perceptions we are working with, as illustrated in Example 4.2.

Example 4.2: The different meanings of an art group

Mr Jones was detained in hospital, during an episode of hypomania, after getting involved with the police when he threatened a checkout girl in a local supermarket. While on ground leave with the occupational therapist, he refused to return to the ward and held on to a lamp post, shouting for help. Following this incident, his leave was suspended until his mood stabilized.

When well, Mr Jones was an enthusiastic amateur painter. In order to help him cope with the frustration of not being allowed to leave the ward, the occupational therapist attempted to engage him in a twice-weekly art group. Mr Jones was offended by the poor quality of materials available to the group but believed that he had to attend as a condition of having his leave restored. The occupational therapist thought that the painting group had a positive meaning for Mr Jones, while he saw it as an unpleasant task that had been imposed on him.

There is a sense in which an occupation belongs to the person who engages in it and puts her own meaning into it, as illustrated in Example 4.3. A piece of performance can be experienced as a task, rather than an occupation, if the individual does not feel that sense of ownership, perhaps because someone in authority has told her to do it.

Example 4.3: Ownership of an occupation

Naomi is known in the village for her beautiful garden, which she cares for herself. Gardening is an important occupation for her because it gives her pleasure, organizes a large part of her time and contributes to her social identity and status.

Following a fall, Naomi has to move to sheltered housing, where the garden is cared for by a paid gardener. Naomi is no longer able to carry out the activities she used to do in her own garden but gardening remains one of her occupations. She discusses garden design with the gardener, makes suggestions about appropriate plants and is writing a book on organic pest control. Her activities associated with gardening have changed but it remains one of her main occupations.

The ownership is of the gardening, not of the garden, so that Naomi is still able to experience it as an occupation even when she does not have her own garden and cannot carry out gardening activities herself.

A specific action carried out at a particular time may be perceived as an occupation, an activity or a task depending on various personal and contextual factors. In other words, the terms do not refer to the action itself but to how the performer conceptualizes it, as explained in more detail in the next section.

Shifting perspectives

In Chapter 3, we looked at some of the dimensions of doing that change the perspective of the performer: meaning–no meaning, observable–non-observable, physical environment–sociocultural environment, spatiotemporal dimension–no spatiotemporal dimension, whole–part and complex–simple. As explained in the last section, these dimensions influence whether a piece of performance is experienced as an occupation, an activity or a task. These shifts of perspective depend on the context in which the task, activity or occupation is performed and the meaning that the individual gives to what she or he is doing, which is, in turn, influenced by the context. For example, a person watching television might experience it as an activity, as leisure or as doing nothing. This could depend on whether he has chosen to watch television on that occasion or if it is a default activity because he cannot think of anything more interesting to do.

The meaning that a piece of performance has for the performer may change each time it is carried out. For example, whether or not a woman experiences cooking as an occupation or an activity depends partly on the meaning that it holds for her on the particular occasion when she is doing it. If she is cooking a meal because she loves trying out new recipes and enjoys serving good food to her partner, this is an occupation for her. If she is not interested in cooking but has to produce a meal for the family because her partner works full time, she may perceive cooking as an activity or a task.

Meanings can also change during a piece of performance, so that what is experienced at one moment as an activity becomes an occupation at another point in the process. Finally, the nature of what we do changes over the course of our lives, so that what is an activity for a child might become an occupation for an adult.

It is possible to experience something as an occupation even when some of the activities that contribute to the occupation are experienced as negative. Pleasure is not the only dimension that gives meaning to an occupation or activity. For example, Mike experiences sitting an examination as an unpleasant experience but he will do it because it contributes to an occupation that he values, that of studying for a degree. For Mike, sitting the examination is not an end in itself but is an essential part of being a student.

If the negative meanings of an activity or occupation outweigh the positive ones, the performer will experience occupational alienation and may become ill if he does not perform the activity differently or do something different.

A piece of performance can be perceived by the performer as complete in itself or may be seen as contributing to a greater whole. Depending on the context, the same piece of performance may shift from being a task to an activity to an occupation and back again, as shown in Example 4.4.

Example 4.4: Shifting perspectives between task, activity and occupation

Jennifer is an occupational therapist who writes and edits occupational therapy textbooks. Sometimes she sees herself as an occupational therapist who writes textbooks and sometimes as a writer who practises occupational therapy. When she thinks of occupational therapy as her main work occupation, Jennifer perceives authoring a textbook as an activity and writing as one of the tasks which make up that activity. When she thinks of editing and writing textbooks as her main work occupation, Jennifer experiences writing as an activity.

In this section we have considered some of the ways in which the relationships between terms can change, so that the conceptual framework is not a static structure but a dynamic way of conceptualizing the complexity of occupation. The definitions of terms remain constant but a piece of performance can be experienced as an occupation, an activity or a task depending on the perspectives of the performer.

SUMMARY

This chapter discussed in depth the three terms used by occupational therapists to refer to forms of action: *occupation, activity* and *task*. It looked at the common usage of the terms and the ways that they are used by occupational therapists. The European definition of each term was given, with an explanation of how the definition was constructed and what it means. The final section of the chapter explored the relationships between the three terms.

The next chapter discusses another cluster of terms from the action interface: the action cluster.

REFERENCES

College of Occupational Therapists (2004) *Occupational Therapy Standard Terminology Project Report.* London: College of Occupational Therapists.

College of Occupational Therapists (2006) *Recovering Ordinary Lives: The Strategy for Occupational Therapy in Mental Health Services, a Vision for the Next Ten Years.* London: College of Occupational Therapists.

Creek, J. (1998) 'Purposeful activity.' In J. Creek (ed.) *Occupational Therapy: New Perspectives.* London: Whurr.

Creek, J. (ed.) (2002) *Occupational Therapy and Mental Health, Third Edition.* Edinburgh: Churchill Livingstone.

Creek, J. (2003) *Occupational Therapy Defined as a Complex Intervention.* London: College of Occupational Therapists.

Creek, J. (2008) 'The knowledge base of occupational therapy.' In J. Creek (ed.) *Occupational Therapy and Mental Health, Fourth Edition.* Edinburgh: Churchill Livingstone.

Cullen, A. (2005) 'Weathering winter woes.' *Healthy Way 38,* 4, 8–9.

Department of Health (2004) *At Least Five a Week: Evidence on the Impact of Physical Activity and Its Relationship to Health. A Report from the Chief Medical Officer.* London: Department of Health.

Forsyth, K. and Kielhofner, G. (2006) 'The model of human occupation.' In E.A.S. Duncan (ed.) *Foundations for Practice in Occupational Therapy, Fourth Edition.* Edinburgh: Elsevier.

Fortmeier, S. and Thanning, G. (2002) *From the Patient's Point of View.* Copenhagen: Danish Association of Occupational Therapists.

Friedland, R.P., Fritsch, T., Smyth, K.A., Koss, E., *et al.* (2001) 'Patients with Alzheimer's disease have reduced activities in midlife compared with healthy control-group members.' *Proceedings of the National Academy of Sciences 98,* 6, 3440–3445.

Golledge, J. (1998) 'Distinguishing between occupation, purposeful activity and activity, Part 1: review and explanation.' *British Journal of Occupational Therapy 61,* 3, 100–105.

Hagedorn, R. (2000) *Tools for Practice in Occupational Therapy: A Structured Approach to Core Skills and Processes.* Edinburgh: Churchill Livingstone.

Harvey, A.S. and Pentland, W. (2004) 'What do people do?' In C.H. Christiansen and E.A. Townsend (eds) *Introduction to Occupation: The Art and Science of Living.* Upper Saddle River, NJ: Prentice Hall.

Iwama, M.K. (2006) *The Kawa Model: Culturally Relevant Occupational Therapy.* Edinburgh: Churchill Livingstone Elsevier.

Lavin, B. (2005) 'Occupation under occupation: days of conflict and curfew in Bethlehem.' In F. Kronenberg, S.S. Algado and N. Pollard (eds) *Occupational Therapy without Borders: Learning from the Spirit of Survivors.* Edinburgh: Elsevier.

Long, C. (2004) 'On watching paint dry: an exploration of boredom.' In M. Molineux (ed.) *Occupation for Occupational Therapists.* Oxford: Blackwell.

McDonald, R., Surtees, R. and Wirz, S (2004) 'The International Classification of Functioning, Disability and Health provides a model for adaptive seating interventions for children with cerebral palsy.' *British Journal of Occupational Therapy 67,* 7, 293–302.

New Shorter Oxford English Dictionary (1993) Oxford: Clarendon Press.

Polatajko, H.J., Davis, J.A., Hobson, S.J.G., Landry, J.E., *et al.* (2004) 'Meeting the responsibility that comes with the privilege: introducing a taxonomic code for understanding occupation.' *Canadian Journal of Occupational Therapy 71,* 5, 261–264.

Smith, H.C. (2005) '"Feel the fear and do it anyway": meeting the occupational needs of refugees and people seeking asylum.' *British Journal of Occupational Therapy 68,* 10, 474–476.

Social Exclusion Unit (2004) *Mental Health and Social Exclusion: Social Exclusion Unit Report.* London: Office of the Deputy Prime Minister.

Wanless, D. (2004) *Securing Good Health for the Whole Population: Final Report.* London: HM Treasury.

Wenborn, J. (2005) 'Making occupation matter for older people in care homes.' *British Journal of Occupational Therapy 68,* 8, 337.

World Health Organization (2001) *International Classification of Functioning, Disability and Health.* Geneva: World Health Organization.

CHAPTER 5

ACTION

INTRODUCTION

The last chapter explored the meanings of three key terms used in occupational therapy to refer to professional purpose and practice: *occupation*, *activity* and *task*. The meanings of these terms and the relationships between them were discussed, focusing on how these relationships change depending on the perspective of the performer and the context of the performance.

This chapter will extend our understanding through a detailed exploration of the four terms in the cluster of action: *occupational performance*, *activity performance*, *task performance* and *occupational performance areas*.

OCCUPATIONAL/ACTIVITY/TASK PERFORMANCE

This section explores the common understanding of *performance* and then looks at how occupational therapists have combined it with *occupation*, *activity* and *task* to create a specialized terminology for doing. Where a lay person might talk about working, playing, sleeping or cooking, an occupational therapist brings all these doing words together under the umbrella of performance.

What occupational/activity/task performance mean in common usage

Unlike the terms in the first chapter, those defined in this chapter are not used outside occupational therapy. In everyday language, the word *performance* is rarely heard used in conjunction with *occupation* or *activity*: these are specialist terms that have been coined by occupational therapists. However, it is more common to hear the phrase *task performance*, as in 'She performed her daily tasks cheerfully', although people may also talk about task accomplishment.

The *New Shorter Oxford English Dictionary* (1993) offers three definitions of *performance*:

1. The execution or accomplishment of an action, operation or process undertaken or ordered; the doing of any action or work; something performed or done; an action, a deed.

2. The carrying out or fulfilment of a command, duty, purpose, promise etc.

3. The action of performing a play, a part in a play, a piece of music etc.

Performance is commonly used in the first sense when talking about the success of a business or enterprise. So, we read about the performance of a chain of high street shops over the first quarter of the year, or about the performance of the chief executive of a company. We talk about good performance and poor performance. The concept of performance is widely used by health and social care providers in relation to meeting targets and staying within budgets. Performance indicators are objective markers that can be used to demonstrate whether or not an individual or organization is meeting its goals.

Performance is used in the second sense to refer to some aspects of what people do, for example, we may hear about a police officer being killed in the performance of his duties. The word may also be used to refer to the tasks carried out by non-human entities, so we can talk about the performance of a new computer or discuss a high-performance car engine.

The word is used in its third meaning when we talk about drama or live music, which are often referred to as performance arts. We may read the review of a new performance of *The Tempest* by the Royal Shakespeare Company, or refer to someone who reads his work in public as a performance poet. A display of exaggerated behaviour or unnecessary fuss may also be called a performance.

In everyday speech, people discriminate between the things that they do by using more precise words than performance. Someone might say that she 'is *studying* for a European Computer Driving Licence at evening classes', or that she '*went shopping* at the weekend for an outfit to wear at a friend's wedding', or that she '*had to walk* to work on Wednesday because there was a bus drivers' strike'. All these phrases refer to what occupational therapists would call *occupational performance, activity performance* or *task performance.*

The World Health Organization (2001) *International Classification of Functioning, Disability and Health* (ICF), which was developed as 'a standardized and common language permitting communication about health and health care across the world' (p.3), refers to task execution and activity execution. Execution is given two qualifiers: performance and capacity. Performance is 'what an individual does in his or her current environment' (p.15) and capacity is the 'individual's ability to execute a task or an action' (p.15). This means that an individual's performance may be limited by his environment, even when he has the capacity to execute a particular activity.

How occupational therapists use the terms

Occupational therapists define *performance* in a way that is close to the first meaning in the *New Shorter Oxford English Dictionary*. For example, a British occupational therapist, Mary Roberts, wrote that performance

> is the process or manner of functioning, which incorporates what a person does and how it is done. Performance is the outward expression of skills [and] the degree to which an individual is competent, that is, whether there is achievement or failure in doing an activity. (Roberts 2002, p.276)

This section discusses the ways that occupational therapists use the three phrases: *occupational performance, activity performance* and *task performance.*

OCCUPATIONAL PERFORMANCE

When occupational therapists attach the word *performance* to occupation, activity or task, they are using it in the first sense given in the *New Shorter Oxford English Dictionary*: the doing or accomplishment of any action or work. So, *occupational performance* refers to the active, or doing, aspect of occupation; *activity performance* refers to the doing aspect of activity, and *task performance* is the doing aspect of a task.

In the 1980s, occupational therapists began to develop models for practice based on their own theories, rather than drawing on medical or psychological theory. Two American occupational therapists, Reed and Sanderson (1980), published a book in which they described some of the models being explored at that time and emphasized the centrality of the concept of occupational performance in occupational therapy thinking.

Another American, David Nelson (1988), further explored the idea of occupational performance, asserting that occupation can be defined un-ambiguously as the relationship between occupational form and occupa-tional performance. Occupational form is the sociocultural and physical characteristics of the occupation, its physical environment and human con-text. Nelson (1988, p.634) wrote that performance means 'to go through or carry out something' and that occupational performance means 'to go through or carry out the occupational form'. So, occupational perform-ance is what an individual does in carrying out an occupation.

In the late 1980s, a Canadian occupational therapy task force de-veloped a model of occupational performance, based on Reed and Sanderson's work (Sumsion and Blank 2006). In this model, occupational performance is described as an interaction between the capabilities of the individual and factors beyond the individual, such as her or his develop-mental level and the environment (Law *et al.* 1994). The authors empha-sized that occupational performance is 'defined by each individual, based on his or her experience rather than on objective observations' (p.4).

In 1997, two Australian occupational therapists, Chapparo and Ranka, published a Model of Occupational Performance (Australia), which ex-tended the concept of performance 'beyond "doing" to incorporate "knowing" and "being", concepts fundamental to humanism' (Chapparo and Ranka 2005, p.62). In this model, occupational performance is not simply the action component of occupation but incorporates motivation and purpose. This conceptualization comes closer to the European defini-tion of occupational performance, which includes the word 'choice'.

The UK definition of occupational performance in the occupational therapy standard terminology (College of Occupational Therapists 2004) includes both the idea of interaction with the environment and the con-cept of choice: 'occupational performance is interaction of the individual with the environment through the selection, planning and carrying out of activities that contribute to occupations and roles' (*ibid.*, p.2).

Occupational therapy intervention can be targeting at different levels of performance, such as the three levels of functioning described in the ICF (World Health Organization 2001): body structures and functions, activity and participation. Occupational therapists intervene at all three levels but the goals they set at the lower levels are intermediate steps on the way to achieving participation through occupation. For example, an occupational therapist might assist the client to manage his panic attacks (*body function*) so that he is able to do his own shopping (*activity*) as a step towards living independently in his own flat (*participation/occupation*). If the overall purpose of occupational therapy intervention is to facilitate occupation and participation, then the aspect of occupational performance that is of most concern is not the client's observable actions but the accomplishment of occupational goals.

ACTIVITY PERFORMANCE

In the 1990s, occupational therapists began to reclaim the word *occupation* to refer to our professional purpose and the word *activity* fell into disrepute. For example, Ilott (1995, p.297) suggested that there is an 'increasing interest in and understanding of humans as occupational beings [therefore] the time is right to replace the word "activity" with others that capture the complexity of occupation'.

As the word *activity* came to be used less and less, so there are few examples of the term *activity performance* in the occupational therapy literature. In the United Kingdom definition of occupational therapy as a complex intervention, Creek (2003, p.33) defined activity as 'any mental or physical action that is performed voluntarily'. Roberts (2002, p.276) used the word performance to refer to the level of 'achievement or failure in doing an activity' but did not use the phrase activity performance. Similarly, Hagedorn (2001, p.166) defined performance as 'engagement in a task or activity'. She also defined occupational performance as 'the act of engagement in…occupations and daily activities' (*ibid.*, p.5), thus contributing to the conceptual confusion between occupation and activity.

If the occupational therapist in clinical practice chose to use the term *activity performance*, she would be referring to how someone carries out a particular activity, such as cooking a meal – including what she cooks, her method of cooking, how frequently she cooks a meal and how well she does it.

TASK PERFORMANCE

As described in Chapter 4, many occupational therapists think of tasks and activities being located within a hierarchical relationship; for example, a task is 'a constituent part of an activity' (Creek 2002a, p.588). Task performance is, therefore, a component of activity performance. However, Hagedorn defined a task as 'a self-contained piece of performance with a completed purpose or product' (Hagedorn 2000, p.311).

An alternative definition of task is: 'both serious and playful situations for performance in the environment' (Kielhofner 1992, p.159). In this conceptualization, a task sets the requirements for performance so that different tasks require people to perform in different ways.

The phrase *task performance* is used in the context of the cognitive disabilities model (Allen 1985), for example, 'our patients' diseases cause restrictions in task performance' (p.5). In this model, the cognitive dimensions of task performance are described as 'attention, behavior, purpose, experience, process, and time' (Kielhofner 1992, p.109).

Although the phrase *task performance* is found more frequently in the occupational therapy literature than *activity performance*, the most frequently used term remains *occupational performance*.

How occupational/activity/task performance are understood within the conceptual framework

The European definitions of *occupational, activity* and *task performance* were constructed from existing definitions of the terms, using the method described in Chapter 1:

. . . .

Occupational performance is choosing, organizing and carrying out an occupation in interaction with the environment.

. . . .

. . . .

Activity performance is choosing, organizing and carrying out an activity in interaction with the environment.

. . . .

. . . .

Task performance is choosing, organizing and carrying out a task in interaction with the environment.

. . . .

These definitions were constructed from five elements found in the literature in definitions of occupational, activity and task performance. The elements of performance are the same in each definition: only the action being performed is different. The elements are:

• choosing

• organizing

• carrying out

• occupation, activity or task

• in interaction with the environment.

There are three stages in performing an occupation, activity or task: choosing, organizing and carrying out. These are usually performed in sequence, although there will be some overlap during most occupations, activities or tasks. For example, I choose to have a cup of tea and begin organizing the necessary materials and utensils. During this process, I make further choices about what type of tea to use, whether to have it in a mug or a cup, where to drink it and so on. I start the process of making tea with a choice, and then choice, organization and action overlap and interact while I am performing the activity.

All occupations, activities and tasks are performed within interacting environments that influence both the process and the experience of performance. These include physical, social, cultural, political, economic and temporal environments. For example, I can make a cup of tea in my own kitchen more easily than in someone else's kitchen because I am familiar with the physical environment. If I am making a cup of tea for someone else, the process may be punctuated by asking that person what type of tea she or he prefers, how strong, with or without milk and in a cup or a mug. On a Sunday morning, I may make a pot of tea and take it back to bed for a leisurely start to the day. On a working morning, I may opt for a tea bag in a mug as I hurry to get ready before leaving the house to catch my bus. The concept of *environment* is discussed in Chapter 11.

The extent to which a piece of performance is experienced as task, activity or occupational performance depends on an interplay between personal factors and sociocultural factors, as illustrated by Example 5.1.

Example 5.1: Occupational, activity or task performance?

Jennifer, Johanna and Miguel jointly wrote a paper for a conference but had to decide who would present it. Jennifer often speaks at conferences and thought of presenting the paper as the performance of a familiar activity. Miguel could only get funding to attend the conference if he presented a paper, so he saw this as the performance of a task that would contribute to his career as an occupational therapy academic. Johanna loves communicating with others and saw this as an opportunity to perform one of her most valued occupations.

In the last section, we looked at how the term *occupation*, and hence *occupational performance*, has been brought back into use by occupational therapists in the last 20 years, with a concurrent decline in the use of the words *activity* and, to some extent, *task*. The European conceptual framework gives different meanings but equal value to all three words, as discussed in Chapter 3.

The next section looks at how occupational performance can be perceived as falling into different categories or performance areas.

OCCUPATIONAL PERFORMANCE AREAS

The phrase *occupational performance areas* was coined by occupational therapy theorists and is not used or understood outside the profession of occupational therapy. The *New Shorter Oxford English Dictionary* (1993) defines an area as 'a field..., a range of topics, scope, extent'. This means that an occupational performance area, as understood by occupational therapists, is a field of occupation encompassing a range of activities. Examples of occupational performance areas are paid employment, active leisure and household management. For example, one of Cathy's occupations is needlework which, for her, is in the occupational performance area of leisure. Cathy's needlework activities include dressmaking, mending, making soft furnishings and embroidery.

In common usage, people sometimes refer to a field of occupation, for example, 'I work in the field of leisure'. Although most people would not use the term *occupational performance area*, they are aware that their lives encompass different fields of activity, such as work and leisure, and would be able to say which field a particular activity fell into, if asked. Perceptions of leisure may be influenced by a person's age; for example, an older person might think that leisure means idleness and believe that it is not good to be idle.

Activity performance and task performance are not divided into performance areas. The performance of an activity or task can contribute to many different occupations and occupational performance areas, sometimes simultaneously.

How occupational therapists use the term occupational performance areas

Occupational performance areas are categories of occupational performance. For example, the Canadian Model of Occupational Performance (CMOP) suggested three performance areas: self-care, productivity and leisure (Canadian Association of Occupational Therapists 1993). Self-care occupations include personal care occupations, such as grooming and physical fitness, and community living occupations, such as household management and shopping. Productivity occupations include education, unpaid homemaking and paid work. Leisure occupations include recreation, entertainment and using community resources.

From this categorization, we can see that occupations do not fit neatly into occupational performance areas. For example, household management comes into the category of self-care while homemaking is a productivity occupation.

There is no universal agreement on the areas that occupational performance can be divided into, or even on how many areas. For example, in the UK, Creek (2002b) offered the same categories as those in the CMOP: self-care, play/leisure and productivity/work, while Hagedorn (2001) suggested that occupations can be analysed into work, leisure or activities of daily living. In the USA, Christiansen and Baum (1997) described four types of occupation: work; play or leisure; self-maintenance or self-care, and sleep. However, the American Occupational Therapy Association (2002) used the same three categories as Hagedorn: activities of daily living; work and productive activities, and play or leisure activities. Two North American occupational therapists, Christiansen and Townsend (2004), suggested 11 categories of occupation: housework; leisure; recreation; play; study, including apprenticeship and training; sleep and rest; relaxation; sports; travel; retirement, and personal care.

The classification of occupational performance areas is a common-sense categorization, not a scientific one, and few theorists explain why they have chosen the categories that they use. Christiansen and Townsend (2004) identified several ways in which occupations can be classified or grouped:

- according to their purpose or goal, for example, maintaining the living environment or earning money. The goals of occupation may be interpersonal, personal achievement or pleasure

- according to what is done

- according to where it is done

- according to how they are accomplished.

Hagedorn (2001, p.41) pointed out that 'the therapist's traditional division of occupations into work, leisure or activities of daily living must be acknowledged as artificial [because] classification is contextual – what one person regards as a chore may be a hobby for someone else'. She also acknowledged that a particular piece of occupational performance might fit into different categories: for example, making a dress can be a paid job (productivity) for a seamstress, an activity of daily living (self-care) for a woman who cannot afford to buy new clothes, and a hobby (leisure) for a teenager who enjoys designing her own clothes.

A piece of occupational performance can be perceived as moving from one category to another, or being in more than one category at the same time, for the same person, depending on the context. For example, a woman making a dress for her daughter to wear at the school disco might think of this as an enjoyable activity that they can share (leisure) or, if she is very busy and has to sew late at night in order to get the dress finished in time, she might see it as a necessary chore (productivity). She might even see making the dress from both perspectives so that it is categorized simultaneously as leisure and productivity.

While it is the perception of the performer that determines which occupational performance area an activity fits into, most people do not think about their activities in this way: occupational performance is a concept used by the therapist rather than by the client. Categorizing occupations into performance areas is useful to the therapist in several ways. Hagedorn (2001) wrote that it allows the therapist to assess what sort of balance there is between the performance areas in a person's life. For example, does a man work long hours and have little time to spend with his family? Does an unemployed person feel that he does not have any leisure activities because his time is not structured by work?

How the term occupational performance areas is understood within the conceptual framework

The European definition of *occupational performance areas* was constructed from elements found in existing definitions:

· ·

Occupational performance areas are categories of tasks, activities and occupations that are typically part of daily life. They are usually called self-care, productivity and leisure.

· ·

This definition is made up of three elements:

• categories of tasks, activities and occupations

• typically part of daily life

• usually called self-care, productivity and leisure.

Occupational therapists categorize different areas of occupational performance and give names to them, such as work, play or study. Tasks, activities and occupations can all be classified in this way.

These categories of performance are typically part of everyday life, in that they cover the things people do every day. An individual's life is likely to be filled by tasks, activities and occupations that can be categorized in one or more of the three areas of self-care, productivity and leisure. These areas have been given the same labels as the categories of occupation discussed in Chapter 4.

Some occupations are difficult to fit into this system of classification because they are only performed in exceptional circumstances. For example, after a major disaster such as the 2004 tsunami in Asia, the main occupation for many people becomes survival, as they struggle to meet their basic needs. Self-care, productivity and leisure occupations are subsumed into the overarching occupation of survival.

The names given to the areas of occupational performance areas are not definitive. As described in the previous section, occupational performance can be grouped in several alternative ways (Christiansen and Townsend 2004).

Just as a piece of performance can be viewed as a task, an activity or an occupation, depending on the context and the perspective of the performer, so a piece of occupational performance can be perceived as fitting within one area on one occasion and in a different area on another occasion. These shifts of perspective are discussed further in the next section.

RELATIONSHIPS BETWEEN THE TERMS REPRESENTING ACTION

The word *performance*, which is the term that occupational therapists use to refer to doing, or action, is in the centre of the conceptual framework because what people do is the main focus of our interventions:

> The main long-term outcome goal of occupational therapy is for the client to achieve a satisfying performance and balance of occupations, in the areas of self care, productivity and leisure, that will support recovery, health, well being and social participation. (Creek 2003, p.32)

Chapter 4 described how occupation, activity and task are differentiated in the mind of the person carrying out the actions, rather than the difference being apparent to the observer. Similarly, a piece of performance is perceived by the individual as occupational, activity or task performance, based on how she or he experiences it, as illustrated by Example 5.1.

A particular piece of performance can be experienced differently by the individual on different occasions, or even change in the mind of the performer while it is occurring, as shown in Example 5.2.

Example 5.2: The changing meaning of performance

Sylvie had to study gardening when she was an occupational therapy student but did not enjoy it. For her, working in the college garden was the performance of a task that contributed to her occupation of being a student. Now, she has her own garden and takes great pleasure in growing both flowers and vegetables: gardening has become the performance of an occupation.

Just as a piece of performance can be experienced as occupation, activity or task, so a piece of occupational performance can be perceived as self-care, productivity or leisure, or even as belonging in more than one category at the same time, as illustrated in Example 5.3.

Example 5.3: Occupational performance areas

When Sylvie digs her vegetable patch she is aware that the physical exercise is good for her health and well-being (self-care), she plans to grow enough onions and garlic to provide for all her needs this year (productivity) and she enjoys spending her spare time out in the open air after working indoors all week (leisure).

Shifting perspectives

Some of the dimensions of performance that help us to understand how it can be experienced as occupation, activity or task are the meanings that the performance has for the individual, the environment in which it takes place and the degree of complexity involved.

The meaning of what someone does is never fixed or absolute. We cannot say that a performance has meaning or it has no meaning: there are levels or degrees of meaning and this influences how the performer perceives what she or he is doing. This is illustrated in Example 5.4.

Example 5.4: Finding meaning in everyday activities

Two months after her 17-year-old son was killed in a road traffic accident, Mrs Green took an overdose of painkillers in attempt to take her own life. She was found by her husband and admitted to hospital. When she returned home, the community occupational therapist visited her. Mrs Green said she now realized that her husband and their married daughter would be devastated if she died, so she was determined not to make another suicide attempt. However, all her usual activities had lost their meaning so that it seemed pointless to do anything.

The occupational therapist suggested that it was to be expected that Mrs Green would think of her daily activities as chores or duties that had to be done, but she should also try to find some activities that she was able to enjoy. Together, Mrs Green and the therapist produced a short list of pleasurable activities, such as taking a warm bath, working on a patchwork quilt that she was hand-stitching, and going shopping with her daughter. Mrs Green agreed to spend time on at least one of these activities every day.

Mrs Green continued to do the necessary household chores and began to look forward to the pleasurable activities she did every day. Gradually, she found that housework was no longer such an effort and she could once more take pride in making a beautiful home.

One element that gives meaning to a performance is having choices about what to do, but the level of choice involved in task performance is different from that involved in activity performance. The performance of a task contributes to the performance of an activity, therefore the way that the task is performed is constrained by the activity of which it is a part. For example, threading a needle is one of the tasks involved in hand sewing and my choices of needle and thread are determined by what is to be stitched. If I am going to darn a sock, the thread will be darning wool and the needle will be a darning needle. If I am doing bead weaving, the yarn will be a fine multifilament thread and the needle will be a long, slender beading needle. I have a choice about what activity to perform, but once that choice is made it limits my choice of tasks.

The environment also contributes to determining whether performance is experienced as occupation, activity or task. Occupational performance takes place within a social and cultural context that shapes how it is done. For example, parenting is modified by the expectations and norms of the culture in which it takes place:

> Although U.S. middle-class adults often do not trust children below about age 5 with knives, among the Efe of the Democratic Republic of Congo, infants routinely use machetes safely... Likewise, Fore (New Guinea) infants handle knives and fire safely by the time they are able to walk. (Rogoff 2003, p.5)

Task performance always takes place in a physical environment: for example, chopping vegetables is done on a board, with a knife or chopper, in a kitchen or other cooking area. Occupational performance may include mental activities, which do not require a physical environment, although the environment may have an influence on the performance, as illustrated by Example 5.5.

Example 5.5: The influence of environment on performance

Kit is an internationally renowned academic. When she is planning a keynote lecture, she thinks about what she wants to say for several weeks, in a variety of locations, before starting to write. She finds walking in the woods particularly conducive to this kind of reflective thought. However, if she wants to think deeply while travelling on a train, she sometimes wears earplugs to cut out the noise of mobile phones and other people's conversations.

Activity performance shares the cultural and social environments of the occupation to which it is contributing, and is shaped by those environments. This means that the performance of an activity will differ when it contributes to different occupations, as illustrated by Example 5.6.

Example 5.6: Activity performance in different occupations

Michelle is a nightclub singer. When she sings with her backing group in a club, she wears outrageous clothes and dances around the stage with the microphone. Michelle is also a committed Christian. When she sings with her church choir, she wears the choir uniform and tries not to stand out. In both instances, Michelle's activity is singing but it is performed as part of two different occupations.

In addition to having social and cultural dimensions, occupational performance usually involves the performance of many tasks and activities, so that it is necessarily more complex than activity or task performance. This is shown in Example 5.7.

Example 5.7: Degrees of complexity in occupational, activity and task performance

In order to perform as a nightclub singer, one of her main occupations, Michelle has to: find suitable songs; practise with her backing group; keep up-to-date with what audiences want; negotiate fees with club managers; choose appropriate clothes to wear; experiment with different styles of make-up; visit the hairdresser regularly; attend dance and keep fit classes; listen to other singers, and so on. The effective performance of this occupation is very complex.

Singing in a club is one of the activities that Michelle performs as part of her occupation of nightclub singer. The performance of this activity involves getting to the club, dressing for her act, singing on stage with her backing group, accepting applause, changing into her everyday clothes and going home. This sequence of tasks is less complex than the many and varied additional activities that are involved in performing as a nightclub singer.

The first task to be performed when singing in a nightclub is to get to the club. Michelle is picked up by one of her backing singers and driven there in her car. The performance of this task is relatively simple compared with the range of performance demands involved in the full activity.

SUMMARY

This chapter discussed the four terms used by occupational therapists to refer to action, or doing: *occupational performance, activity performance, task performance* and *occupational performance areas*. These are specialized terms that are not used or understood by the general public but they are important for our understanding of how people experience the things that they do.

The next chapter discusses a third cluster of terms from the action interface: structuring action.

REFERENCES

Allen, C.K. (1985) *Occupational Therapy for Psychiatric Diseases: Measurement and Management of Cognitive Disabilities.* Boston, MA: Little Brown.

American Occupational Therapy Association (2002) 'Occupational therapy practice framework: domain and process.' *American Journal of Occupational Therapy 56,* 6, 609–639.

Canadian Association of Occupational Therapists, Health Canada (1993) *Occupational Therapy Guidelines for Client-Centred Mental Health Practice.* Toronto: CAOT Publications ACE

Chapparo, C. and Ranka, J. (2005) 'Theoretical contexts.' In G. Whiteford and V. Wright-St Clair (eds) *Occupation in Practice and Context.* Sydney: Elsevier.

Christiansen, C. and Baum, C. (1997) 'Understanding occupation: definitions and concepts.' In C. Christiansen and C. Baum (eds) *Occupational Therapy: Enabling Function and Well-being, Second Edition.* Thorofare, NJ: Slack.

Christiansen, C.H. and Townsend, E.A. (2004) 'An introduction to occupation.' In C.H. Christiansen and E.A. Townsend (eds) *Introduction to Occupation: The Art and Science of Living.* Upper Saddle River, NJ: Prentice Hall.

College of Occupational Therapists (2004) *Occupational Therapy Standard Terminology Project Report.* London: College of Occupational Therapists.

Creek, J. (2002a) 'Glossary of occupational therapy terms.' In J. Creek (ed.) *Occupational Therapy and Mental Health, Third Edition.* Edinburgh: Churchill Livingstone.

Creek, J. (2002b) 'The knowledge base of occupational therapy.' In J. Creek (ed.) *Occupational Therapy and Mental Health, Third Edition.* Edinburgh: Churchill Livingstone.

Creek, J. (2003) *Occupational Therapy Defined as a Complex Intervention.* London: College of Occupational Therapists.

Hagedorn, R. (2000) *Tools for Practice in Occupational Therapy: A Structured Approach to Core Skills and Processes.* Edinburgh: Churchill Livingstone.

Hagedorn, R. (2001) *Foundations for Practice in Occupational Therapy, Third Edition.* Edinburgh: Churchill Livingstone.

Ilott, I. (1995) 'Let's have a moratorium on activities (the word, not the deed).' *British Journal of Occupational Therapy 58,* 7, 297–298.

Kielhofner, G. (1992) *Conceptual Foundations of Occupational Therapy.* Philadelphia, PA: F.A. Davis.

Law, M., Baptiste, S., Carswell, A., McColl, M.A., Polatajko, H. and Pollock, N. (1994) *Canadian Occupational Performance Measure, Second Edition.* Toronto: CAOT Publications ACE.

Nelson, D. (1988) 'Occupation: form and performance.' *American Journal of Occupational Therapy 42,* 10, 633–641.

New Shorter Oxford English Dictionary (1993) Oxford: Clarendon Press.

Reed, K. and Sanderson, S.R. (1980) *Concepts of Occupational Therapy.* Baltimore, MD: Williams & Wilkins.

Roberts, M. (2002) 'Life and social skills training.' In J. Creek (ed.) *Occupational Therapy and Mental Health, Third Edition.* Edinburgh: Churchill Livingstone.

Rogoff, B. (2003) *The Cultural Nature of Human Development.* Oxford: Oxford University Press.

Sumsion, T. and Blank, A. (2006) 'The Canadian Model of Occupational Performance.' In E.A.S. Duncan (ed.) *Foundations for Practice in Occupational Therapy, Fourth Edition.* Edinburgh: Elsevier.

World Health Organization (2001) *International Classification of Functioning, Disability and Health.* Geneva: World Health Organization.

CHAPTER 6

STRUCTURING ACTION

INTRODUCTION

In the last two chapters we looked at the terms occupational therapists use to refer to the things that people do in their daily lives. These terms are organized into two clusters: *forms of action* and *action*. Forms of action are *occupations*, *activities* and *tasks*, and Chapter 4 discussed both the similarities between these terms and why there is practical utility in differentiating between them. Actions are *occupational performance*, *activity performance*, *task performance* and *occupational performance areas*. Chapter 5 explored how people define their own performance and highlighted the importance of the occupational therapist working with people's own definitions and understandings.

Each person's daily life is filled with the performance of occupations, activities and tasks that are organized into patterns to suit the needs of the individual and the demands of his physical and social environments. The American occupational therapist, Hasselkus, described how these patterns create stability and security in the lives of individuals and communities:

> Routines, habits, and rituals offer us sources of cultural stability in an otherwise chaotic existence, and, without these sources of stability, we human beings could not survive... These behavioral patterns are occupations that offer us ways to ensure the presence of and the structure for the 'familiar' in our daily lives. (Hasselkus 2002, p.49)

The purpose of this chapter is to develop an understanding of the terms *habit* and *routine* that make up the cluster: structuring action.

HABIT

The noun *habit* has several meanings in the English language, including: clothing; posture; bodily constitution; characteristic mode of growth; mental disposition; dependency on an addictive drug, and tendency to act in a certain way (*New Shorter Oxford English Dictionary* 1993). This chapter addresses only the last meaning, tendency to act in a certain way, which is the one most relevant to occupational therapy. While occupational therapists also use the word habit in its penultimate meaning, dependency on an addictive drug, this meaning is shared with other health care workers and is not part of the specialized professional vocabulary represented by the European conceptual framework.

What habit means in common usage

The *New Shorter Oxford English Dictionary* (1993) defines *habit* as:

1. A settled disposition or tendency to act in a certain way, *esp.* one acquired by frequent repetition of the same act until it is almost involuntary.

2. A customary practice or way of acting.

In the first sense, we might talk about developing good habits of personal hygiene, or describe nail biting as a bad habit. Although a habit is defined as almost involuntary, there is an implication that the individual can change it if he wants to do so and is prepared to make the effort. In other words, we are responsible for our own habits, good or bad. If someone intends to do something that we disapprove of, such as getting drunk, we might tell her not to make a habit of it, meaning that getting drunk once might not do too much harm but it should not be indulged in regularly.

The second sense of the word is more general: we might say that someone has the habit of finishing other people's sentences for them, or that a miserly person has the habit of leaving the pub before it is his turn to buy a round of drinks. In this sense, a habit expresses something about the person who embodies it; that he is too impatient to let other people finish what they want to say, or that he is too mean to pay for a round of drinks.

One of the ways that people express continuing pleasure in an activity, such as watching the Wimbledon tennis tournament on television, is to say that it is habit-forming. Used in this context, the phrase more often has positive connotations, rather than the negative ones associated with a drug or alcohol habit.

How occupational therapists use the term habit

For the occupational therapist, 'habits are the basic structures by which daily behaviour is ordered in time and psychosocial health is maintained' (Kielhofner 1977, p.239). Occupational therapists are interested in people's habits because of the problems that occur when they fail to develop, develop in a maladaptive way or are disrupted. There are two ways in which habits can become problematic:

- when they are absent or weak, so that the individual's life is chaotic or his thought processes are tied up with thinking about what he is doing. For example, when 'learned behaviours are no longer available through subcortical mechanisms, automaticity is lost, and cortical attention must be utilized in order to perform' (Breines 1981, p.70)

- when they are inflexible, as in obsessive compulsive disorder, so that the individual's time is taken up with activities that do not meet his needs or serve no practical purpose.

An American occupational therapist, Winifred Dunn (2000, p.7S) defined habits as 'patterns of human behavior' and suggested that they can be organized onto a continuum, from habit impoverishment at one end to habit domination at the other, corresponding with the two problems listed above. Habit impoverishment is 'a condition in which habits do not support daily life' and habit domination is 'a condition in which habits or rituals are so demanding that they interfere with daily life' (Dunn 2000, p.7S). In the centre of the continuum is habit utility, 'a condition in which habits or routines support performance in daily life and contribute to life satisfaction' (*ibid,*. pp.7S–8S).

Habits, provided they are not too rigid or too loose, are useful in helping us to organize our lives effectively without having to think all the time about what we are doing. Hasselkus (2002, p.49) described habits as liberating because they 'enable us to live *enriched lives* and to experience enhanced periods of creativity and innovation by the fact that they "free the brain" from the work of attending to the repetitive concerns of people's daily lives'. A similar idea was expressed by Clark (2000, p.129S): 'habit formation may create optimal conditions for functioning creatively, productively, and efficiently'.

Clark and colleagues (2007, pp.15S–16S) identified five advantages of habits:

1. They channel resources in a consistent direction and so minimize incoherence and indecision.

2. They conserve energy by enabling the organism to avoid the constant formation of neural pathways or the need for repeated decision making.

3. They allow more economical speed of action.

4. They use environmental input as a guiding force.

5. They increase skill through repetition and so increase the likelihood of success.

Breines (1986, p.246) defined a habit as 'automatic behaviour which results from repetition, and which is engaged in without conscious attention or awareness'. Once a habit has been established, we can perform it automatically while our thoughts are on other things. For example, I do not have to think about cleaning my teeth in the morning but do it automatically while thinking about how to conduct a meeting or what to buy for dinner.

Clark and colleagues (2007) carried out a review of the literature on habit and identified a number of different ways in which the term has been defined and understood. What all these have in common is that 'habit is construed as a relatively unconscious, nonreflective, and repeatable phenomenon [and] with the exception of tics, habits are also categorically viewed as acquired, although they are seen as linked in certain instances with instinct' (p.15S).

The early occupational therapists were concerned with restoring or establishing good habits in their patients through a technique called habit training:

> Habit training is based on the laws of exercise, frequency and recency and is an attempt to restore or maintain those acquired behaviour patterns which enable us to perform many tasks efficiently and with little or no conscious thought. (Macdonald 1960, p.117)

The concept of habit training has disappeared from the occupational therapy literature but has been replaced by a similar concept, that of habit formation, in lifestyle redesign programmes that are designed and run by occupational therapists (Clark, Jackson and Carlson 2004). Habit formation involves gaining experience in healthy lifestyle practices along with 'a process of self-analysis through which [the participant performs] a personal inventory of...goals, strengths, interests, patterns of activity and weaknesses' (*ibid.*, p.206). These two strands of the lifestyle redesign programme are brought together into customized daily routines that eventually become habits, so that lifestyle changes are sustained.

Another concept similar to habit training is that of habituation or learning through repetition (Rowles 2000). Habituation has been defined as 'an internalized readiness to exhibit consistent patterns of behavior guided by our habits and roles and fitted to the characteristics of routine temporal, physical and social environments' (Kielhofner 2002, p.63).

Confusion between the terms *habit* and *routine* is common in the occupational therapy literature. For example, at an occupational therapy research conference on habit, it was noted that 'participants used the term *habit* synonymously with terms such as *routine, habitual behavior, complex regime,* and *routinization.* Further, participants...lacked consensus on the meaning of habit' (Rogers 2000, p.120S). In attempting to clarify this issue, Clark (2000, p.126S) suggested that 'routines are a kind of habit [but] not all habits are routines'. In a later paper, she classified routine as one category of habit: 'Morning routines, family routines, work procedures, and protocols fall into this category of habit' (Clark *et al.* 2004, p.12S).

Dunn (2000) referred to habits, rituals and routines without distinguishing between them. In the occupational therapy literature, a ritual has been defined as 'a linking of past, present and future...recurrent events that can contain both continuity and change' (Farnworth 2003, p.119). This term does not form part of the European conceptual framework and will not be discussed further in this chapter. The similarities and differences in meaning between *habit* and *routine* are clarified in the conceptual framework. The European definition of *habit* is discussed in the next section.

How habit is defined within the conceptual framework

· ·

A *habit* is a performance pattern in daily life, acquired by frequent repetition, that requires minimal attention and allows efficient function.

· ·

This definition was constructed from five elements found in existing definitions of *habit* in the occupational therapy literature:

- performance

- pattern in daily life

- acquired by frequent repetition

- requires minimal attention

- allows efficient function.

A habit is a way of structuring performance, which might be task performance, activity performance or occupational performance. For example, when Barbara drives her car she does not have to think about how to change gear or stop at the traffic lights: she has been driving long enough for these tasks to have become habits. She is an occupational therapist at a local hospital and always follows the same route to work, without having to think about it: the activity of driving to work has become a habit. Barbara works from nine to five, Monday to Friday so she does not have to plan when to go to work: her paid work occupation has become a habit.

Habits structure performance into patterns that make sense to people and give shape to their daily lives. For example, Mike walks his dog on the beach for an hour every morning and evening, whatever the weather. He loves the companionship of his dog and, since retirement and the death of his wife, he has planned all his other activities around their daily walks.

For an action to become a habit, it has to be practised or carried out until it becomes automatic. Frequent repetition of a sequence of actions performed in the same way each time produces the automatic performance that forms a habit. When Barbara first learned to drive a car, she had to concentrate on all the tasks to be carried out, using hands, feet and eyes. After enough practice, she found that all these actions had become habits so that her driving is now automatic and she can think about other things at the same time.

The performance of a habit requires minimal attention because it is automatic. When Barbara is driving, she pays attention to the road and the driving conditions but does not have to pay attention to what her hands and feet are doing. If there is an emergency, requiring her to brake suddenly, she will do this automatically, despite much of her attention being elsewhere.

Developing many of our predictable daily actions into habits enables us to function efficiently because we can pay most of our attention to any unpredictable events or complex situations that need to be addressed.

ROUTINE

We have already identified that occupational therapists sometimes use the words *habit* and *routine* synonymously, but clarifying the differences between the two terms has practical value, as will be explained in this section.

What routine means in common usage

The *New Shorter Oxford English Dictionary* (1993) defines *routine* as:

1. A regular course of procedure.

2. An unvarying performance of certain acts.

3. Regular or unvarying procedure or performance.

In the first sense, we might say that the security checks at an airport departure gate are a routine, because they are always carried out in the same way with all passengers. We might also talk about a novelist having a routine of getting to his desk by 8 a.m. and writing for six hours every day. This meaning of the word does not carry positive or negative connotations; it is just how things are done.

In the second sense, we might say that someone becomes irritable when her daily routine is disrupted, meaning that she likes to do the same things, in the same order, at the same time every day. In this sense, routine comes closer to the meaning of habit, with the implication that there is choice involved in an unvarying performance of this sort.

In the third sense, someone might say that he has chosen to work freelance because he would not enjoy the routine of a nine-to-five job. There is a slightly negative connotation in this use of the word, implying that a routine is either not necessary or is boring. The phrase 'a break in routine' is used to refer to a welcome break, such as a holiday, from regular activities that have become dull through repetition.

How occupational therapists use the term routine

Hagedorn (2000) offered two definitions of *routine* that are similar in meaning to the Oxford Dictionary definitions: 'an automated and habitual chain of tasks with a fixed sequence' (p.311) and 'habitual and fixed sequences of activities' (p.26). Hagedorn placed routines in her analytical taxonomy of occupation (see Figure 4.1), between occupations and activities.

Clark (2000, p.127S) suggested a different way of understanding routine, as 'a structure through which occupation is organized'. She also suggested that 'occupations (both habitual and non-habitual), in turn, can be thought of as the building blocks of one kind of routine, daily routines' (p.127S).

Daily routines serve an important purpose in assisting people to organize and manage all the tasks and activities that have to be accomplished in a normal day. For example, a study of mothers caring for children with disabilities observed that they coped better once they were able to establish practical routines for home management and child care: 'the development of workable routines fosters mothers' sense of competence and control' (Larson and Zemke 2003, p.88).

The term temporal adaptation is sometimes used in connection with routine:

> The term *temporal adaptation* is used to refer to the normal use of time in a purposeful daily routine of activities... The healthy individual has his daily life activities organised into a satisfying and flexible pattern that meets his needs and is socially acceptable. Some routines are repeated in the same way until they become habitual and do not require conscious thought. (Creek 2008, p.42)

Parkinson (2004, p.97) advised that occupational therapists need to 'be skilled at advising and coaching individuals regarding the benefits of structure and routine, as we cannot rely on this being self-evident'. Drawing on the work of Kielhofner (2002), she suggested that routines are important for five reasons:

1. They meet our basic biological and psychological needs by providing regularity and predictability.

2. They enable complexity and creativity.

3. They are important for society because they allow us to fit in with others.

4. They contribute to roles, which are built up of interwoven routines.

5. They can assist in overcoming illness.

The next section looks at how *routine* is defined in the European conceptual framework.

How routine is understood within the conceptual framework

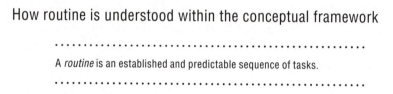

A *routine* is an established and predictable sequence of tasks.

This definition was constructed from three elements found in existing definitions of *routine* in the occupational therapy literature:

• established

• predictable

• sequence of tasks.

A sequence of tasks does not become a routine until it is established; that is, the manner in which it is performed is made stable and secure. Some routines are established by guidelines or protocols, such as the procedure for dispensing medication on an inpatient unit. Other routines are worked out by the individual through trial and error to suit his circumstances and needs. For example, a new mother has to establish a routine that will both meet the needs of her baby and accommodate her other occupations.

A routine is predictable because it always consists of the same tasks carried out in the same sequence. Any variation in either the tasks or the sequence can be described as a disruption of routine. The sudden onset of illness, or an accident, can disrupt a person's normal daily routines, making life unpredictable and insecure.

A routine consists of a number of tasks that are performed in sequence. The sequence may be quite short, for example, checking that all the ingredients are available before starting to make a cake, or longer, as in the sequence of checks that have to be carried out before an aircraft takes off. Any activity can be seen to consist of a series of tasks but it is only described as a routine if the sequence of tasks is unvarying. As discussed in Chapter 4, the sequence of tasks that makes up an activity can be varied in several ways without disrupting successful performance of the activity.

RELATIONSHIPS BETWEEN THE TERMS REFERRING TO STRUCTURING ACTION

The two terms in the structuring action cluster, *habit* and *routine*, are close in meaning and, as identified above, are often used synonymously by occupational therapists. The similarities are in the predictability of the way that actions are performed, which frees the performer from having to think consciously about what is being done. The main difference between the two concepts is that a habit requires minimal attention while a routine, although it is established and predictable, may still require the performer to think carefully about what is being done. For example, when the ground and flight crews are carrying out checks on an aircraft, they perform them in an established sequence but have to pay full attention to what they are doing in order to ensure that no potential problems are overlooked. In contrast, cleaning one's teeth is a habit for most people, so that they can think about other things during the activity.

There is a practical value for occupational therapists in clarifying the difference between habits and routines because either or both can be disrupted and, before intervention can take place, it is necessary to identify exactly what the problem is. Example 6.1 describes how both habits and routines had to be re-established following a house move.

Example 6.1: Re-establishing habits and routines

Mrs Fairweather has been blind since sustaining a traumatic brain injury in her teens. With the assistance of a guide dog, she is independent in personal care, household management and mobility within her local community. When her husband was promoted, the family moved to a new house in a different town.

Following the move, Mrs Fairweather found that all her daily tasks and activities were disrupted, as her habitual ways of doing things did not work in the new house. For example, until she relearned where things were stored in the kitchen, she had to think consciously about where to find them and then where to put them away after use. After a few weeks, as Mrs Fairweather became accustomed to the layout of her new kitchen, she was able to re-establish a set of habits that made her daily chores much easier.

In the old neighbourhood, Mrs Fairweather and the dog had established a routine for doing the shopping that took them past all the necessary shops in the same order each day. They began by walking through a park so that the dog could have a run off the lead and then crossed a busy road at a set of traffic lights, which brought them into a pedestrianized shopping precinct. After the move, Mrs Fairweather enlisted the help of the occupational therapist working for a local charity for people with visual impairment. Together they worked out a routine for doing the shopping that Mrs Fairweather found comfortable, although she now had to give the dog his run on a separate outing. Until the new routines were established, both Mrs Fairweather and the dog were anxious when they had to go out without the therapist but, eventually, they settled happily into their new life.

Shifting perspectives

Whether a sequence of actions is experienced as a habit or a routine can change, depending on the perspective of the performer. For example, a routine may be established by a protocol, such as the hand-washing protocol for infection control. A new nurse, who is learning the routine, has to think about it in order to make sure that he does not miss any steps in the sequence. After a few weeks on the ward, the routine becomes a habit that he performs without conscious thought.

The meaning of both habits and routines comes from their familiarity and from the structure that they bring to our lives, although both can be performed without any conscious awareness of their meaning. It is also possible for a habit or routine to have meaning on one occasion and not on another, or for the meaning to change as the context changes, as illustrated by Example 6.2.

Example 6.2: The changing meaning of a routine

When Florence gets home from work she always puts her briefcase down in the hall, changes into casual clothes and then sits on the settee for half an hour with a glass of wine. This routine represents a transition from her demanding job to the relaxation and freedom of being at home. On the day that Florence received an important promotion, she followed her usual routine but its meaning had changed and the glass of wine became a toast in celebration of her success.

The meaning of a routine may also be different from the perspectives of the performer and the observer, as in Example 6.3.

Example 6.3: Performer and observer interpretations of routine

Mr Stead, a 32-year-old computer programmer, has a volitional disorder and has great difficulty in carrying out a range of necessary or expected daily activities, such as housework. In consequence, his house is extremely dirty. The community occupational therapist is encouraging him to establish a daily cleaning routine that will ensure a basic standard of hygiene in his living environment. She is the observer of Mr Stead's housekeeping routines.

In her own home, the occupational therapist has a much more flexible routine for housework because household chores have to be fitted around her other commitments. Rather than doing the same tasks at the same time every week, she not only chooses when to carry out her household duties but also decides how thoroughly she will do them.

The therapist's interpretation of the nature and purpose of routine changes, depending on whether she is an observer or a performer.

Both habits and routines are performed within a physical environment. Habits are usually more personal than routines, which often have a sociocultural dimension. For example, Joaquim has the habit of turning the light out whenever he leaves a room but, in his job as departmental manager, he is expected to follow a routine for checking that all the equipment and lights have been turned off before he leaves.

A habit may be one part of a routine in which other tasks are not habits, as shown in Example 6.4.

Example 6.4: One part of a routine becoming a habit

Florence does not think about putting her briefcase down in the hall when she gets home: the action is a habit. However, although changing her clothes is another part of her homecoming routine, she does not always change into the same clothes. If friends are coming to dinner she will wear a pretty dress but if she plans to do some gardening after her drink she will put on a pair of jeans.

Both habits and routines can be either simpler or more complex, as illustrated by two habits in Example 6.5.

Example 6.5: Simple and complex habits

Stephanie works as a pharmacist in a chemist's shop in the next street to her house. The simple journey from her front door to the shop takes less than five minutes to walk and she does this automatically: walking to work is a habit.

Jennifer regularly travels to London as part of her job, entailing a five-hour journey from door to door. Despite the complexity of taking a bus, two trains and the London underground, she usually performs the journey without thinking about the sequence of actions. For example, at the departure station she automatically goes to the right platform and, on arrival at her destination in London, she automatically walks to the appropriate exit from the underground. Unless the journey is disrupted by external circumstances, she experiences this complex five-hour journey as a habit.

This section has explored the relationship between the two terms in the structuring action cluster, showing how a sequence of actions can be perceived as either a *habit* or a *routine*, or as a mixture of the two.

SUMMARY

This chapter explored the terms used by occupational therapists to refer to the ways that people structure their actions: *habit* and *routine*. It looked at how these terms are used by the general public and in the occupational therapy literature. The European definitions of both terms were given, with explanations of how the definitions were constructed and what they mean. The final section considered the relationship between the two terms, highlighting the dynamic nature of that relationship.

The next chapter looks at the fourth and final cluster of terms in the action interface of the conceptual framework: *boundaries to action*.

REFERENCES

Breines, E. (1981) *Perception: Its Development and Recapitulation*. Lebanon, NJ: Geri-Rehab Inc.

Breines, E. (1986) *Origins and Adaptations: A Philosophy of Practice*. Lebanon, NJ: Geri-Rehab Inc.

Clark, F.A. (2000) 'The concepts of habit and routine: a preliminary theoretical synthesis.' *Occupational Therapy Journal of Research (Supplement)*, 20, 123S–137S.

Clark, F.A., Jackson, J. and Carlson, M. (2004) 'Occupational science, occupational therapy and evidence-based practice: what the well elderly study has taught us.' In M. Molyneux (ed.) *Occupation for Occupational Therapists*. Oxford: Blackwell.

Clark, F.A., Sanders, K., Carlson, M., Blanche, E. and Jackson, J. (2007) 'Synthesis of habit theory.' *OTJR: Occupation, Participation and Health Vol. 27, Supplement*, 7S–23S.

Creek, J. (2008) 'The knowledge base of occupational therapy.' In J. Creek and L. Lougher (eds) *Occupational Therapy and Mental Health, Fourth Edition*. Edinburgh: Churchill Livingstone.

Dunn, W.W. (2000) 'Habit: what's the brain got to do with it?' *Occupational Therapy Journal of Research (Supplement)*, 20, 6S–20S.

Farnworth, L. (2003) 'Time use, tempo and temporality: occupational therapy's core business or someone else's business.' *Australian Occupational Therapy Journal*, 50, 116–126.

Hagedorn, R. (2000) *Tools for Practice in Occupational Therapy: A Structured Approach to Core Skills and Processes*. Edinburgh: Churchill Livingstone.

Hasselkus, B.R. (2002) *The Meaning of Everyday Occupation*. Thorofare, NJ: Slack.

Kielhofner, G. (1977) 'Temporal adaptation: a conceptual framework for occupational therapy.' *American Journal of Occupational Therapy 31*, 4, 235–242.

Kielhofner, G. (2002) *A Model of Human Occupation: Theory and Application, Third Edition*. Baltimore, MD: Lippincott Williams & Wilkins.

Larson, E.A. and Zemke, R. (2003) 'Shaping the temporal patterns of our lives: the social coordination of occupation.' *Journal of Occupational Science 10*, 2, 80–89.

Macdonald, E.M. (1960) *Occupational Therapy in Rehabilitation: A Handbook for Occupational Therapists, Students and Others Interested in This Aspect of Reablement*. London: Ballière, Tindall & Cox.

New Shorter Oxford English Dictionary (1993) Oxford: Clarendon Press.

Parkinson, S. (2004) 'The importance of routine in acute mental health settings.' *Mental Health Occupational Therapy 9*, 3, 97–98.

Rogers, J.C. (2000) 'Habits: do we practice what we preach?' *Occupational Therapy Journal of Research (Supplement), 20*, 119S–122S.

Rowles, G.D. (2000) 'Habituation and being in place.' *Occupational Therapy Journal of Research (Supplement), 20*, 52S–67S.

CHAPTER 7

BOUNDARIES TO ACTION

INTRODUCTION

The cluster of terms used to refer to the boundaries to action is the last cluster in the interface between the internal and external worlds of the occupational being. Chapter 6 looked at how people structure their actions into *habits* and *routines*: this chapter explores the boundaries that define and shape action.

The cluster consists of four terms: *autonomy, dependence, independence* and *interdependence*. Together, these terms explain the conditions under which an individual is able to act freely and independently and the importance of social and physical environments as barriers to or facilitators of action.

The concepts of *dependence* and *independence* have always been important for occupational therapists but this does not mean that they have been well understood or unproblematic. An example of the problematic nature of the concept of independence was highlighted by an American occupational therapist, Betty Hasselkuss, when she said that the rehabilitation ideology of independence has been a source of tension in occupational therapists' understanding of relation: 'Relation is being *with* others, feeling connected with one's world; independence is acting *without* others, functioning separately from others, using personal initiative' (Hasselkuss 2002, p.94).

In recent years, the notion of *interdependence* has become more widely used and this term helps to highlight the problematic nature of our understanding of dependence and independence.

In the UK, the Mental Capacity Act (2005) presented a set of principles to be followed when considering whether or not to deprive someone of their right to *autonomy*. People with some form of mental disorder, such as a mental health condition, a brain injury or a learning disability, must be assumed to be able to make their own decisions unless it is established that they lack capacity. Furthermore, all practicable steps should be taken to help people to make their own decisions for as long as they are capable of doing so: depriving someone of their autonomy is a last resort.

AUTONOMY

In societies that place a high value on individual freedom and independence, autonomy is seen as a virtue: 'to be deficient in autonomy is to be too dependent on the support, prompting and advice of others' (Benson 1983, pp.5–6). The autonomous individual is a free agent who can rely on his own powers in forming opinions, choosing and acting. He 'has a mind of his own and a will of his own. He exercises independence in his thinking and in his decisions about practical affairs' (*ibid.*, p.6).

What autonomy means in common usage

In the *New Shorter Oxford English Dictionary* (1993) *autonomy* is defined in five ways, as:

1. The right or condition of self-government.

2. Freedom of the will.

3. Independence.

4. Freedom from external control or influence.

5. Personal liberty.

The first sense of the word is used when we say that the government of China has established several national autonomous regions, such as Xinjiang Uygur province, that are accorded cultural autonomy although they do not have political freedom. This means that they have the right to determine their own cultural practices.

We are using autonomy in its second sense when we say that someone has exercised her autonomy, meaning that she has used the freedom to follow her own chosen course of action.

When autonomy is used in the sense of independence, we might say, for example, that learning to drive will give a young person greater autonomy.

In the fourth sense of the word, we might talk about a unit manager having the autonomy to make decisions without prior reference to central management.

Using autonomy in the sense of personal liberty, we might say that women are given less autonomy in some cultures than in others. The Chilean economist Max Neef (1991) wrote of autonomy being one of the conditions that can satisfy the human need for freedom.

The moral philosopher Seedhouse (1988, p.130) defined autonomy as: 'a person's capacity to choose freely for himself, and to be able to direct his own life'. He pointed out that 'autonomy is hardly ever pure but restricted by factors such as the law, social tradition, the autonomy of other people, and the prevailing circumstances of a person's life' (p.130).

The concept of autonomy is of great importance in the field of medical ethics, given that doctors sometimes have to make decisions that will affect the lives of people whose autonomy is compromised by illness or unconsciousness. The moral philosopher O'Neill (1984, p.173) pointed out that 'autonomy is lacking or incomplete for parts of all lives (infancy, early childhood), for further parts of some lives (unconsciousness, senility, some illnesses and mental disturbance) and throughout some lives (severe retardation)'.

Autonomy is highly valued in those societies where the individual is seen as the social unit, rather than the family or the community. This carries the concomitant expectation that people will make their own choices and that those choices will be responsible. Benson (1983, p.8) said that there is 'a kind of autonomy which is a much more basic virtue, namely the willingness to undertake for oneself the ordinary tasks of daily life'.

How occupational therapists use the term autonomy

Occupational therapists use the word *autonomy* far less often than the related term, *independence*, when talking about their clients. However, it has begun to appear more frequently in the occupational therapy literature in recent years, perhaps due to an increased interest in the concept of client-centred practice (Parker 2006). For example, an occupational therapist working in a forensic setting carried out a small study into the impact of a client-centred approach on the autonomy of male offenders (Morrow 2008). The definition of autonomy that she chose to use was one appropriate to her study population: 'being responsible for oneself, for one's deeds and development' (Rogers 2002, cited in Morrow 2008, p.35).

Barnitt (1998) carried out a study in which therapists were asked to tell stories of ethical dilemmas they had experienced at work, which were then analysed for the features of ethical reasoning they demonstrated. One example was 'the strongly argued case for patient/client autonomy as a general ethical principle that should be adopted when working with a patient' (p.88).

Despite this rhetoric of promoting client autonomy and giving patients choices about their treatment, there is often still an expectation that people will choose to do what the staff consider to be good for them. Hagedorn (1995, p.53) wrote of a social contract in which society 'protects the rights of the individual to do as he wishes, while imposing upon him constraints and responsibilities'. The occupational therapist has to balance the principle of promoting individual autonomy against the duty to protect the client and others against the consequences of socially unacceptable choices.

Creek (1998, 2007) developed a theory to explain the interactions between motivation, volition and autonomy during engagement in activity. She drew on the work of Raanon Gillon (1985, 1986), a moral philosopher who suggested that there are three types of autonomy (Creek 2007, p.134):

1. autonomy of thought: being able to think for oneself, to have preferences and to make decisions

2. autonomy of will: having the freedom to decide to do things on the basis of one's deliberations

3. autonomy of action: the capacity to act on the basis of reasoning.

Creek (2007) warned that autonomy can be compromised by personal circumstances, environmental barriers or social pressures. Hagedorn (1995, p.53) suggested that 'autonomy [is not] a stable concept, for expectations vary according to an individual's age, sex, culture, role and responsibilities'.

Occupational therapists are not only concerned about their clients' autonomy but also about their own autonomy. For example, Jenkins (1998, p.42) wrote about the importance of enabling 'partnership and participation without compromising either professional or client autonomy'. However, Barnitt, in an unpublished paper delivered at the World Federation of Occupational Therapists Congress in 1994, pointed out that constraints and restrictions placed on the therapist's autonomy can interfere with her ability to promote client autonomy. Barnitt also highlighted that it is not always possible to respect both client autonomy and therapist autonomy when their choices are incompatible. An example of such a conflict is given in Example 7.1.

In the European conceptual framework, the concept of autonomy refers to the experience of the performer, whether that is the client exercising autonomy in the performance of his occupations or the therapist exercising autonomy in her practice.

Example 7.1: Conflict between client and therapist autonomy

An occupational therapist, Sarah, believed that promoting client autonomy was an essential aspect of client-centred practice and a central part of her role. When a client was unable to make autonomous decisions, Sarah would make an assessment of the problem and incorporate the development of autonomy as a goal of intervention.

John had a mild stroke after the death of his wife and was referred to Sarah for help with managing his domestic activities and increasing his social contacts. As part of the initial assessment, Sarah asked John what he saw as his main problems and what he would like to achieve. John thought that Sarah, as the professional, should be able to carry out an assessment and tell him what his problems were. He also expected her to advise him on which problems should be tackled first and what the most appropriate intervention would be.

Sarah's preferred course of action was incompatible with what John wanted and expected of her. In order to respect his autonomous decision to delegate decisions about treatment to her, Sarah had to put her own preferences to one side.

How autonomy is used within the conceptual framework

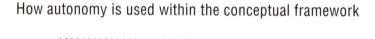

Autonomy is the freedom to make choices based on consideration of internal and external circumstances and to act on those choices.

This definition was constructed from four elements taken from existing definitions in the occupational therapy literature:

- freedom to make choices

- internal circumstances

- external circumstances

- freedom to act.

As pointed out earlier in this chapter, autonomy is not an all-or-nothing concept. The freedom to make choices may be compromised by personal circumstances, such as illness, or by social or environmental constraints. However, most people experience some degree of freedom of choice at some times in their lives.

The concept of autonomy is based on the assumption that people are able to make rational choices that take account of their circumstances. However, autonomy is never absolute but is always partial and specific to a particular situation: it may be compromised by internal or external circumstances. It is neither rational nor useful to make choices that cannot be enacted because of internal or external constraints. For example, René enjoys skiing but he does not choose to ski every weekend because the nearest ski slopes are several hundred miles from where he lives.

Internal circumstances that might have to be considered when making choices include state of health, knowledge of own capabilities and awareness of the consequences of a particular choice. External circumstances that might have to be considered when making choices include environmental supports and barriers, social expectations and competing demands.

It is possible to make a free choice but not have the freedom to act on that choice, due to internal or external factors. Internal factors that can compromise autonomy include fear, ignorance and passivity and external factors include oppression and lack of resources (Max Neef 1991). For example, Jane decided to have a day out in London on her birthday but rail services were disrupted by snow and she was unable to get there. Her autonomy was compromised by adverse weather conditions.

DEPENDENCE

Dependence is often seen by occupational therapists as a deficiency and the concept is not widely used: therapists prefer to focus on independence, which is generally seen as a positive attribute. A South African occupational therapist, Nicholls (2007), pointed out that everyone is, to some extent, dependent on others but most people prefer to deny that dependence. She suggested that cultural assumptions about interdependence tend to reinforce the hatred of dependence.

What dependence means in common usage

In English, the term *dependence* is used in several ways, including the action of hanging down, subjection or subordination and the condition of waiting in faith or expectation. These meanings of the word are not addressed here. Other definitions of *dependence* are (*New Shorter Oxford English Dictionary* 1993):

1. The relation of having existence hanging upon, or conditioned by, the existence of something else.

2. The fact of depending *on* another thing or person.

3. The state or condition of being dependent.

4. The condition of a dependant.

5. Inability to do without someone or something.

In the first sense of the word, we might talk about the dependence of the Yorkshire fishing fleets on stocks of fish in the North Sea. If fish stocks fail, the fleets will not survive.

The word is being used in its second sense when we refer to the dependence of a young child on his mother or the dependence of an elderly person on his walking frame. There are different types of dependence: for example, the child's dependence on his mother is both emotional and physical; the elderly man's dependence on his walking frame is mainly physical.

In order to understand the concept of dependence in its third sense, we have to look at definitions of *dependent* (*New Shorter Oxford English Dictionary* 1993):

1. Contingent on or determined or conditioned by something else.

2. Resting entirely on someone or something for maintenance, support, or other requirement.

3. Unable to do without someone or something.

In this sense, then, dependence is the state or condition of being determined by something else, of resting entirely on someone or something for a requirement or requirements or of being unable to do without some-one or something. So we might say that a couple have to place their de-pendence on the estate agent to sell their house after they move overseas, or that a woman's dependence on her mother's help increased after the birth of her third child.

In order to understand the fourth meaning of dependence, we have to look at definitions of *dependant*. A dependant is 'a person who de-pends on another for maintenance or position' (*New Shorter Oxford English Dictionary* 1993). So, dependence in this sense means the condition of depending on another for maintenance or position, as when a wife gives up work after the birth of her first child and accepts financial dependence on her husband.

The last sense of *dependence* is similar to the first sense, so we might talk about an Afghan farmer's total dependence on the income from his opium crop, or the dependence of a person with pernicious anaemia on regular injections of B12.

How occupational therapists use the term dependence

As stated at the beginning of this section, occupational therapists rarely write about the concept of *dependence*. However, three conceptualizations can be found in the occupational therapy literature: dependence as a prob-lem, dependence as rewarding, and dependence as a desirable attribute.

DEPENDENCE AS A PROBLEM

Nicholls (2007) suggested that occupational therapists and other health care staff may deny the need for dependence in themselves and others as a defence against vulnerability. She argued that dependence on others is both 'a necessary and problematic part of us' and that 'each person must struggle with feelings of dependency on others' (Nicholls 2007, pp.61–62).

DEPENDENCE AS REWARDING

It has been suggested that dependent behaviours can, in certain situations, lead to social interaction, such as the interactions between paid carers and residents of nursing homes. 'The dominant response by institutional staff to a resident's independent behaviors is no response; independent behav-iors do not generate social interactions' (Hasselkuss 2002, p.94). In such situations, dependence brings the reward of social interaction.

DEPENDENCE AS A DESIRABLE ATTRIBUTE

A Japanese–Canadian occupational therapist, Michael Iwama, has argued that occupational therapists' attitudes to dependence are culturally determined. In Japan, he says, dependence in social relationships is both normal and healthy (Iwama 2006). The Japanese word for this social dependence is *amae*, which means 'the need of an individual to be loved and cherished; the prerogative to presume and depend upon the benevolence of another' (Doi 1971, in Iwama 2006, p.27).

How dependence is used within the conceptual framework

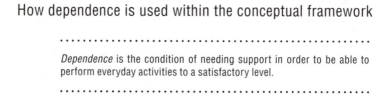

Dependence is the condition of needing support in order to be able to perform everyday activities to a satisfactory level.

This definition was constructed from four elements found in definitions of dependence taken from the occupational therapy literature:

- condition
- needing support
- to perform everyday activities
- satisfactory level.

A condition is a state or mode of being, for example, the phrase 'health condition' is often used to refer to the state of a person's health. So the condition of dependence refers to the state or extent of a person's reliance on external support.

To need support is to require help, assistance or services, which may be of different types such as practical, financial or emotional. We might say that a visually impaired student needs (practical) support to find his way around the university library, or that he needs (financial) support from his parents while he is studying, or that he needs extra (emotional) support from his girlfriend when taking examinations.

The concept of performing everyday activities is a familiar one to occupational therapists. Activity performance was defined in Chapter 5 as choosing, organizing and carrying out activities in interaction with the environment. Everyday activities are all the things that people do in their daily lives, including work activities, play, social activities, personal care and domestic activities. Each person has a range of everyday activities that he expects to perform on a regular basis.

What constitutes a satisfactory level of performance is determined by the performer and will vary from one person to another. Personal standards are influenced by social standards and social expectations, so the satisfactory level is constituted through interplay between the individual and the social context. This means that what is considered satisfactory in one context may be unsatisfactory in another, as illustrated in Example 7.2.

Example 7.2: What is a satisfactory level of performance?

Felix and Elliot are taking a creative writing course together. Felix thinks that being able to express his ideas eloquently is the most important aspect of his work and he does not worry if he makes spelling mistakes or grammatical errors. Felix's tutors do not penalize him for grammatical errors, because they want to encourage his creativity, but when he submits a short story to a magazine he has to make sure that it is written in good English.

Elliot also wants to be able to communicate his ideas fluently but he is offended by what he considers to be poor grammar or faulty spelling and he is careful to check all his coursework for errors.

INDEPENDENCE

Independence tends to be highly valued in Western society, in theory if not always in practice. It is acceptable for young children, seriously ill or severely disabled people and those who are both elderly and infirm to be dependent on others but everyone else is expected to achieve, or at least to strive for, the greatest possible degree of independence.

What independence means in common usage

The word *independence* is given two meanings in the English language (*New Shorter Oxford English Dictionary* 1993):

1. The condition or quality of being independent.

2. An income sufficient to relieve one from the need to earn one's living.

The meaning of *independent* is related to definitions of *dependent*. To be independent means (*New Shorter Oxford English Dictionary* 1993):

1. Not subject to the authority or control of any person, country etc.

2. Free to act as one pleases.

3. Autonomous.

4. Not dependent or contingent on something else for its existence, validity, effectiveness etc.

In its first meaning, *independence* is the condition or quality of not being subject to authority or control, free to act as one pleases, autonomous or not dependent on something else for existence, validity or effectiveness. We are using the word in this sense when we talk about a war of independence or about a young person reaching the age of independence at 18. We might say that not having to go to work on a public holiday gives a welcome sense of independence, or a newly divorced woman might feel that she has regained her independence. We sometimes differentiate between different types of independence, such as financial independence or emotional independence.

The term is being used in its second sense when we say that someone has inherited an independence from his uncle, or that a life insurance policy will provide a widow with an independence rather than a fortune.

Various forms of independence are highly valued in Western society, both in the sense of not being subject to control and of being financially viable. For example, Lim and Iwama (2006, p.168) felt that Western societies strongly value personal autonomy and independence, in contrast to some non-Western cultures that 'focus more on collective interest and agreement'.

How occupational therapists use the term independence

The concept of *independence* is an important one within occupational therapy but Wilcock (2002) found that it was first officially used in relation to activities of daily living in a government publication of 1955: *Services for the Disabled*. This document stated that 'one of the first essentials of rehabilitation is that the disabled should be as independent as possible in the personal activities of daily living' (quoted in Wilcock 2002, p.264). By the 1970s, Wilcock claimed, the role of the occupational therapist working in social services was largely focused on prescribing equipment to help people to remain independent.

Nicholls (2007, p.79) agreed that 'occupational therapists tend to see the main goal of their work as promoting independence' and to believe that all their clients 'have a desire for self-efficacy and independence'. However, she did not see this goal as entirely legitimate but described it as 'a symptom of the profession's unconscious defense against vulnerability' (*ibid.*, p.79).

Hasselkuss (2002) thought that the goal of independence was a social one, which has been taken up by occupational therapists and other rehabilitation professionals:

> In our social culture, we admire the person who works hard, who doesn't give up, who overcomes obstacles by persistence and 'stick-to-it-iveness.' In the context of rehabilitation, these ideologies are reproduced as goals for individual independence in the everyday activities of life and as expectations for patient behaviors that reflect individual initiative, personal responsibility, and perseverance. (pp.93–94)

Independence is seen by disability activists as the exercise of autonomy across all areas of life but it is sometimes reduced by occupational therapists to independence in activities of daily living (Taylor 2001). This narrow conceptualization shapes how occupational therapists work with their clients, focusing on functional tasks and personal skills, 'often excluding or ignoring the quality, for the disabled individual, of the independent existence' (p.246).

A three-year longitudinal study of occupational therapy students in the UK found that the students' conceptualizations of independence changed and developed throughout their undergraduate years (Taylor 2001). The findings illustrate a disconnection between the rhetoric of occupational therapy, which states that its professional purpose is to give clients choice and control, and what is often done in practice, which is to focus on developing or retraining self-care skills, whether or not the client thinks this is a priority.

Hagedorn (1995, p.53) differentiated between autonomy and independence, as the terms are used by occupational therapists:

> Therapists tend to speak of a person as 'autonomous' when in fact they mean 'capable of exercising choice and control over one's personal life', and as 'independent' when they mean 'able to do what is required to remain healthy, without needing someone else to help'.

This distinction is compatible with the European definitions of autonomy and independence.

How independence is used within the conceptual framework

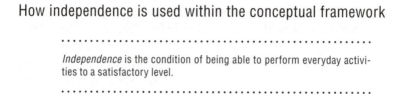

Independence is the condition of being able to perform everyday activities to a satisfactory level.

This definition was constructed from three elements that were taken from existing definitions of the term and from definitions of *dependence* found in the occupational therapy literature. Definitions of both terms were analysed so that the definitions of *dependence* and *independence* would be congruent:

- being able to perform
- everyday activities
- satisfactory level.

By taking elements from existing definitions of both dependence and independence, the working group were able to ensure that consensus definitions of the two terms are compatible. While *independence* is the condition of being able to perform everyday activities to a satisfactory level, *dependence* is the condition of needing support in order to achieve this. The three elements of the definition of *independence* are, therefore, discussed above, in the section on *dependence*.

INTERDEPENDENCE

As highlighted in the introduction, the concept of *interdependence* has become more widely used by occupational therapists in recent years although, like independence, it is understood in different ways.

What interdependence means in common usage

The concept of *interdependence* has come into common use relatively recently. The word is not found in the 1993 edition of the *New Shorter Oxford English Dictionary* and only the adjective, *interdependent*, appears in the 2002 edition.

The *Shorter Oxford English Dictionary* (2002) defines *interdependent* as 'dependent on each other'. As a noun, *interdependence*, therefore, means the state or condition of being dependent on each other. The term cannot be used of an individual because interdependence is a relationship between at least two people or things. For example, there is an interdependence between Lincolnshire potato farmers and the seasonal migrant workers who pick their potatoes.

The development of complexity theory across a range of disciplines has raised awareness of the unpredictable ways in which different parts of a complex system can affect each other. The wide use of this theory may be partly responsible for an increased social understanding and acceptance of the interdependence between people, and between people and the natural world.

How occupational therapists use the term interdependence

Increasing use of the term *interdependence* by occupational therapists has accompanied their changing perceptions of what it means to be independent:

> The more recent rehabilitation literature has questioned the wisdom of declaring independence as an absolute goal in rehabilitation... The term 'interdependence' communicates that those in societies depend on collaboration and cooperation, and that no community dwelling individual is truly independent. (Baum and Christiansen 1997, p.35)

Two North American occupational therapy authors made a distinction between interdependence and mutual dependence:

> Interdependence is a fundamental experience in shared occupations... the expression and satisfaction of being and doing with others. Mutual dependence, sometimes referred to as codependence, may negatively draw people into collusion in harmful occupations. Examples are... codependent families caught up in alcohol, drug, gambling, or other addictions. Positive interdependence, however, generates mutual aid and reciprocal giving. (Christiansen and Townsend 2004, p.145)

Christiansen and Townsend (2004, p.146) took an idealistic view of interdependence, describing it as the foundation for building communities in 'a spirit of social inclusion, mutual aid, and a moral commitment and responsibility to recognize and support difference'.

Iwama (2006) also saw interdependence as a desirable condition but argued that it is more characteristic of Japanese society than Western society. He asserted that Japanese people value 'belonging, interdependence and group harmony', in contrast to Western people who 'may come across as being individualistic, egocentric and self-assured' (Iwama 2006, p.81).

It is possible to include both independence and interdependence as legitimate concerns of occupational therapy. Creek (2008) suggested that occupational therapists may work towards the goals of independence, interdependence or even dependence, depending on the wishes of the client:

> It is possible to make autonomous decisions without compromising healthy interdependence. For example an individual with severe physical disabilities may take the decision to be dependent on others for his self-care so that he can put his energy into pursuing an interesting career. (Creek 2008, p.43)

How interdependence is used within the conceptual framework

· ·

Interdependence is the condition of mutual dependence and influence between members of a social group.

· ·

This definition was written to be compatible with the European definitions of *dependence* and *independence*. It was constructed of four elements from the definitions of *interdependence* that were found in the occupational therapy literature:

- condition

- mutual dependence

- mutual influence

- members of a social group.

As explained in the section on *dependence*, a condition is a state or mode of being; for example, we might say that an athlete needs to be in peak condition to take part in a major competition.

Christiansen and Townsend (2004, p.145) defined interdependence and mutual dependence differently, seeing interdependence as a positive condition, found in healthy communities, and mutual dependence as potentially leading to 'collusion in harmful occupations'. In the European conceptual framework, no such distinction is made: mutual dependence is part of the condition of interdependence.

In addition to mutual dependence, interdependence is also characterized by mutual influence. Influence is 'an action exerted...by indirect means by one person or thing on another so as to cause changes in conduct, development, conditions, etc.' (*Shorter Oxford English Dictionary* 2002). Within a group, such as a family or work team, people change each other's conduct by what they do and the ways that they respond to each other. This is different from the changes brought about by the directives of someone in authority in the group, such as a parent or team leader. The difference between mutual influence and leadership is illustrated in Example 7.3.

Example 7.3: Influence and leadership in multidisciplinary team working

Harriet is the occupational therapist in an inpatient rehabilitation unit for people with severe, enduring mental illness. The unit manager wants the multidisciplinary team to adopt a recovery approach to rehabilitation and has arranged for all staff to attend in-service training with a visiting specialist.

Harriet sees the recovery approach as entirely compatible with her occupational therapy orientation and can see many potential roles for herself. These might include: assessing patients' strengths; working with them to increase their capacity for making personal choices; accompanying patients on trips to explore what community resources they might use, and helping patients to develop their skills through engagement in a varied programme of activities.

Other staff within the team also have ideas about what their contribution might be to the establishment of a recovery approach on the unit. One of the nursing assistants is keen to take responsibility for physical fitness activities and has gained an appropriate qualification. The unit manager thinks that nursing staff should be involved in taking patients on social outings and family visits, if they need an escort. The psychologist feels that she can make an important contribution to assessment.

As Harriet develops her role on the unit, what she does is shaped by both the leadership of the unit manager, who expects her to adopt the recovery approach, and the influence of her colleagues, who are simultaneously developing their own roles.

There are different types of interdependence, such as the interdependence of symbiotic organisms or the interdependence of bees and flowers. The European conceptual framework is concerned with people, so this definition refers to interactions between members of a social group. People naturally participate in a variety of social groups during their lifetimes:

Participation in groups is essential to participation in life. We are born into families, neighbourhoods and communities. As children, we interact in play groups, classrooms, sports teams, religious and political groups, charity organisations, informal social groups and extended family groups. As older adults, we find that group status sustains our integrity as others seek our input or advice. (Cole 2008, p.316)

In this conceptualization, interdependence is seen as a natural condition of group membership throughout the life cycle, although the degree and form that it takes might vary at different times.

RELATIONSHIPS BETWEEN TERMS REFERRING TO THE BOUNDARIES TO ACTION

This detailed analysis of the meanings of terms in the cluster of boundaries to action has shown that each term can only be understood in relation to the others. If a person has a greater degree of independence, he will have less dependence. In order to promote interdependence, an individual may have to give up some of her autonomy. None of the terms represents an absolute condition; that is, no one can have absolute autonomy or absolute independence. Every person will at times experience more or less autonomy, more or less dependence, independence or interdependence. The ratio varies at different stages of the life cycle, with children and very old people being expected to have less autonomy and independence than working age adults, in most societies.

Autonomy does not depend on a person's level of independence: someone may express a high degree of autonomy despite being dependent on the support of others. For example, Juan has never learned to cook because it is women's work and his generation of Spanish men do not cook. When his wife dies, Juan chooses to go and live with his son and daughter-in-law. He makes an autonomous decision to be dependent on his family rather than learning to cook for himself.

A person may be highly independent but have limited autonomy. For example, Susan earns enough money to afford the necessities of life, including paying a mortgage and remaining free of other debts, but she has no cash left over to indulge in her choice of leisure activities, clothes and so on.

It is possible to have both limited autonomy and limited independence. For example, the person with advanced dementia will find it very difficult to make autonomous decisions and will be dependent on others for support in carrying out many of the activities of daily life.

The degree to which someone is dependent, independent or interdependent is influenced by internal factors, including the personal requisites for action described in Chapter 8: *occupational performance components, function, ability* and *skill*. An example of internal factors affecting someone's independence and autonomy is shown in Example 7.4.

Example 7.4: Internal factors affecting autonomy and independence

Averil is a single mother and a university lecturer. She enjoys her job and gets on well with her colleagues: they form a strong team, supporting each other in both teaching and research. For example, when one of them wants to spend some time collecting data or writing up a project for publication the others will arrange to cover her teaching, on the understanding that each person will receive the same support when needed.

Averil suffers from recurrent episodes of major depression. When she is depressed, she finds all aspects of daily life difficult, due to exhaustion, low mood and a sense of hopelessness. She continues going to work when she has the energy but spends a lot of time in bed when she is not working. She becomes dependent on her mother for child care and household management, and on her colleagues to take over some of the burden of work. She finds it hard to make decisions, even simple ones such as what food to buy. As she descends into a depressive episode, Averil is aware that the interdependence between herself and her family, and between herself and her colleagues, is moving towards greater dependence.

For most of her adult life, Averil has experienced repeated swings between feeling independent and in possession of a high degree of autonomy, which she considers to be her normal state, and feeling hopeless, helpless and dependent on others, which she perceives as the result of illness.

The balance between autonomy, dependence, independence and interdependence is also influenced by external factors, including the social and physical environments described in Chapters 10 and 11. An example of this is given in Example 7.5.

Example 7.5: External factors affecting autonomy and independence

James has never learned to drive: this was an autonomous decision taken when he was a teenager and concerned about environmental issues. He lives in a small town in the Yorkshire Dales, which has no railway station but an excellent bus service. He takes the bus to work in a nearby larger town and uses it to reach the nearest railway station when he wants to travel further.

During a period of economic recession, the bus services during the day are cut from four buses an hour to two, evening services are reduced to one bus an hour and Sunday services are discontinued. Since James works shifts, these changes impact on his ability to get to and from work. He is faced with the choice of using a taxi at times when there is no bus service, accepting lifts from colleagues who live in the same town and also work shifts, or learning to drive and buying a car.

James' independence has been compromised by the reduction in bus services but he is still able to exercise autonomy in deciding how best to manage his changed circumstances.

Shifting perspectives

The four terms in the boundaries to action cluster are all abstract and non-observable. For example, we may assume that someone has made an autonomous decision, but this assumption is based on our observation of actions that we think represent the internal state of autonomy. The person making a choice may be aware of whether or not the choice is autonomous, but that conscious awareness can vary depending on circumstances, as shown in Example 7.6.

Example 7.6: Awareness of autonomy

When Lesley's widowed father has a severe stroke, Lesley chooses to reduce her hours of work so that she can become his chief carer. This decision is taken with the support of Lesley's partner, who understands her wish to enable her father to live at home. Lesley visits every day, assists her father with self-care activities, does the housework and accompanies him to hospital appointments. She feels satisfied that she has made the right choice.

Lesley's father's condition deteriorates over time and Lesley finds herself visiting him at least twice a day, including at weekends. She is permanently tired, she finds it difficult to manage on her reduced income and her partner complains about not seeing her at weekends. Lesley now feels that she is trapped and that her choices are very limited. It is hard for her to remember that she undertook the caring role for her father freely and willingly.

The difference between dependence and independence, as they are defined in the conceptual framework, is one of perception. There are no objective criteria for identifying the point at which one can say that an action is performed independently. For example, should the older person who uses a walking stick when walking out of doors be seen as more dependent than someone who uses a walking pole when hill walking? The older person might fear falling and depend on his stick to give him the confidence to go out. The hill walker might find that the walking pole helps him to walk faster but does not see himself as dependent on it.

On the other hand, the hill walker might be afraid to walk without his pole and the older person might be able to manage without the stick. The degree of dependence each person has on his walking aid depends on the meaning that he gives to it.

As described in the last section, autonomy, dependence, interdependence and independence are always partial and always in flux. For example, we can talk about someone making an autonomous decision but we cannot say that someone is autonomous, because autonomy varies in different circumstances. The same applies to dependence and independence: a person may be dependent on others in certain areas of life but independent in other areas.

SUMMARY

This chapter discussed in depth the four terms used by occupational therapists to refer to the boundaries to action: *autonomy, dependence, independence* and *interdependence*. It looked at the common usage of the terms and the ways in which they are used by occupational therapists. The European definition of each term was given, with an explanation of how the definition was constructed and what it means. The final section of the chapter explored the relationships between the terms and the ways in which those relationships change according to internal and external circumstances.

This is the last chapter in the section describing the interface between the internal and external worlds of the performer. The next chapter discusses a cluster of terms from the internal world: the personal requisites for action.

REFERENCES

Barnitt, R. (1998) 'The virtuous therapist.' In J. Creek (ed.) *Occupational Therapy: New Perspectives.* London: Whurr.

Baum, C. and Christiansen, C. (1997) 'The occupational therapy context: philosophy – principles – practice.' In C. Christiansen and C. Baum (eds) *Occupational Therapy: Enabling Function and Well-being, Second Edition.* Thorofare, NJ: Slack.

Benson, J. (1983) 'Who is the autonomous man?' *Philosophy 58*, 5–17.

Christiansen, C.H. and Townsend, E.A. (eds) (2004) *Introduction to Occupation: The Art and Science of Living.* Upper Saddle River, NJ: Prentice Hall

Cole, M. (2008) 'Client-centred groups.' In J. Creek and L. Lougher (eds) *Occupational Therapy and Mental Health, Fourth Edition.* Edinburgh: Churchill Livingstone Elsevier.

Creek, J. (1998) 'Communicating the nature and purpose of occupational therapy.' In J. Creek (ed.) *Occupational Therapy: New Perspectives.* London: Whurr.

Creek, J. (2007) 'Engaging the reluctant client.' In J. Creek and A. Lawson-Porter (eds) *Contemporary Issues in Occupational Therapy: Reasoning and Reflection.* Chichester: Wiley.

Creek, J. (2008) 'The knowledge base of occupational therapy.' In J. Creek and L. Lougher (eds) *Occupational Therapy and Mental Health, Fourth Edition.* Edinburgh: Churchill Livingstone.

Gillon, R. (1985, 1986) *Philosophical Medical Ethics.* Chichester: Wiley.

Hagedorn, R. (1995) *Occupational Therapy: Perspectives and Processes.* Edinburgh: Churchill Livingstone.

Hasselkuss, B.R. (2002) *The Meaning of Everyday Occupation.* Thorofare, NJ: Slack.

Iwama, M.K. (2006) *The Kawa Model: Culturally Relevant Occupational Therapy.* Edinburgh: Churchill Livingstone Elsevier.

Jenkins, M. (1998) 'Shifting ground or sifting sand?' In J. Creek (ed.) *Occupational Therapy: New Perspectives.* London: Whurr.

Lim, K.H. and Iwama, M.K. (2006) 'Emerging models – an Asian perspective: the Kawa (river) model.' In E.A.S. Duncan (ed.) *Foundations for Practice in Occupational Therapy, Fourth Edition.* Edinburgh: Elsevier Churchill Livingstone.

Max Neef, M.A. (1991) *Human Scale Development: Conception, Application and Further Reflections.* New York, London: Apex.

Mental Capacity Act (2005) London: TSO.

Morrow, T. (2008) 'Can a client centred approach develop autonomy and behavioural change in male offenders attending group activities in forensic environments?' *Mental Health Occupational Therapy 13,* 1, 35–39.

New Shorter Oxford English Dictionary (1993) Oxford: Clarendon Press.

Nicholls, L. (2007) 'A psychoanalytic discourse in occupational therapy.' In J. Creek and A. Lawson-Porter (eds) *Contemporary Issues in Occupational Therapy: Reasoning and Reflection.* Chichester: Wiley.

O'Neill, O. (1984) 'Paternalism and partial autonomy.' *Journal of Medical Ethics 10,* 173–178.

Parker, D. (2006) 'The client-centred frame of reference.' In E.A.S. Duncan (ed.) *Foundations for Practice in Occupational Therapy, Fourth Edition.* Edinburgh: Elsevier Churchill Livingstone.

Seedhouse, D. (1988) *Ethics: The Heart of Health Care.* Chichester: Wiley.

Shorter Oxford English Dictionary, Fifth Edition. (2002) Oxford: Clarendon Press.

Taylor, M.C. (2001) 'Independence and empowerment: evidence from the student perspective.' *British Journal of Occupational Therapy 64,* 5, 245–252.

Wilcock, A.A. (2002) *Occupation for Health, Volume 2: A Journey from Prescription to Self Health.* London: College of Occupational Therapists.

CHAPTER 8

PERSONAL REQUISITES FOR ACTION

INTRODUCTION

This chapter explores the first set of terms that, together with the terms in the energy source for action cluster, make up the internal world of the performer. The terms in the personal requisites for action cluster are *occupational performance components, function, ability* and *skill*. The word *function* is given two distinct meanings within the conceptual framework and both definitions are presented in this chapter.

A requisite is 'a required or necessary thing; a thing needed for a purpose' (*Shorter Oxford English Dictionary* 2002). A requisite for action is a thing necessary for action to take place. Personal means located within the individual; belonging to the person as an individual rather than as a member of a group (*Shorter Oxford English Dictionary* 2002). Personal requisites for action are those attributes of the individual that are necessary for her to be able to take action.

OCCUPATIONAL PERFORMANCE COMPONENTS

The term *occupational performance* was discussed in Chapter 5, where it was defined as choosing, organizing and carrying out an occupation in interaction with the environment. In that chapter, it was explained that the phrase is not found in common usage but is a specialist term coined by occupational therapists. This section will briefly explore the concept of *component* in common usage, look at how occupational therapists use the phrase *occupational performance components* and finish with an explanation of how the term is used in the European conceptual framework.

What components mean in common usage

The term *component* is commonly used in several contexts, such as car mechanics and physics. According to the *Shorter Oxford English Dictionary* (2002), *component* has a number of specialized meanings, including: any of the separate parts of a motor vehicle, machine etc.; each of a set of vectors which when combined are equivalent to a given vector, and each of the constituents of a phase system which together constitute the minimum necessary in specifying the composition of the system. None of these meanings is relevant to the European conceptual framework.

The definition of component that is relevant to this chapter is: a constituent part. For example, we might say that tolerance is an essential component of a successful marriage.

So, if the phrase *occupational performance components* were found in common usage, it would mean the constituent parts of occupational performance.

How occupational therapists use the term occupational performance components

The concept of occupational performance came into regular use in the 1980s, following the publication of the *Guidelines for the Client-centred Practice of Occupational Therapy* (Department of National Health and Welfare & Canadian Association of Occupational Therapists 1983), which presented a model of occupational performance. Although most writers acknowledge that occupational performance is made up of various components, there is little agreement about what these components are.

An American occupational therapist, Mosey (1986), described performance components as part of the domain of concern of the occupational therapist. She defined them as 'the building blocks from which occupational performances are fashioned' (p.8) and listed six components: motor function, sensory integration, visual perception, cognitive function, psychological function and temporal adaptation.

In the UK, Hagedorn (1995, p.300) did not write about occupational performance components but she defined a skill component as 'a single, identifiable, part-skill'. She divided skill components into three categories: sensorimotor, such as sensory integration; cognitive, such as cognitive strategies, and psychosocial, such as intrapersonal skills. She also remarked that 'behaviourists are concerned solely with observable skill, by which they generally mean a component of performance' (*ibid.*, p.61).

Writing about purposeful activity, at a time when this term was still frequently used as an alternative to occupation, Creek (1998) suggested that purposeful activity has five components:

• capacities, such as performance skills and temporal awareness

• volition, including intentions and awareness of performing voluntarily

• purpose, which includes both goals and purpose-in-progress

• meaning

• identity.

With the development of several well-articulated models within the occupational performance frame of reference, such as person-environment-occupation models and the ecology of human performance model, occupational therapists began to use the phrase *occupational performance components* more consistently (Chapparo and Ranka 2005). For example, the Canadian Occupational Performance Model refers to personal performance components and lists these as: physical, mental, sociocultural and spiritual (Canadian Association of Occupational Therapists, Health Canada 1993). A revised version of this model changed the terminology to 'the doing (physical), feeling (affective) and thinking (cognitive) components of the person' (Sumsion and Blank 2006, p.111).

A British occupational therapist, Wilby (2007), warned against a trend in occupational therapy towards focusing on performance to the detriment of performance components. She argued that a sound knowledge of performance components enables the occupational therapist to identify the problems underlying performance deficits and to devise appropriate strategies for intervention.

Other authors have written about occupational performance deficits (for example, Molineux 2004), which are described as risk factors that 'impact on the individual at the level of occupational performance components, such as sensorimotor, cognitive or psychosocial elements of occupational performance' (Cronin-Davis, Lang and Molineux 2004, p.171).

How occupational performance components are understood within the conceptual framework

The European definition of *occupational performance components* was constructed from definitions of the term found in the occupational therapy literature:

· ·

Occupational performance components are abilities and skills that enable and affect engagement in tasks, activities and occupations. These can be categorized as, for example, physical, cognitive, psychosocial and affective.

· ·

This definition is made up of four elements, taken from existing definitions:

- abilities and skills

- enable engagement in tasks, activities and occupations

- affect engagement in tasks, activities and occupations

- can be categorised.

Abilities and *skills* are part of the cluster of personal requisites for action and are defined in this chapter. They are personal characteristics, either innate or developed through practice, that enable and support effective occupational performance. Occupational performance would not be possible without abilities, and effective occupational performance would not be possible without skills, therefore these are the essential components of occupational performance. An illustration of abilities and skills as occupational performance components is given in Example 8.1.

Tasks, activities and *occupations* were defined in Chapter 4. These are three forms of action that enable the accomplishment of goals and that support participation in society. *Engagement* is part of the energy source for action cluster and is defined in Chapter 9. It is a sense of involvement, choice, positive meaning and commitment while performing an occupation or activity. Abilities and skills enable a person to experience engagement in what she is doing and affect the quality of that engagement, as illustrated in Example 8.1.

`Example 8.1: Abilities and skills as components of occupational performance

One of Rachel's leisure occupations is horse riding. She has several abilities that support this occupation, including temporal awareness, physical courage and stamina. She has also developed skills that enable her to be a proficient rider, such as mounting, controlling her horse and maintaining a good seat.

When Rachel was first learning to ride, she had to focus on mounting, controlling her horse and maintaining a good seat. Now that these skills have become habitual, through practice and repetition, she is able to engage more deeply with other aspects of riding, such as her relationship with her horse and exploration of the countryside on horseback.

Occupational therapists categorize the abilities and skills that constitute occupational performance components in order to facilitate identification of problems and to devise appropriate strategies for intervention (Wilby 2007). The four categories given in the European definition are not definitive but are given as an example of such categorization. In practice, an occupational therapist will use a categorization that fits with the frame of reference or model that she is using on a particular occasion.

FUNCTION

The term *function* is used by occupational therapists in two distinct ways and both meanings are given here. First, the common usage of the term is discussed, then examples are given of the ways that occupational therapists use the term and finally the two European definitions are explained.

What function means in common usage

The *Shorter Oxford English Dictionary* (2002) gives several meanings to the noun *function*, including: an order or class of people, a religious ceremony, a formal or important social gathering, any of the basic operations in a computer and a mathematical expression containing one or more variables. Six definitions of function are relevant to this chapter:

1. The activity proper or natural to a person or thing.

2. The purpose or intended role of a person or thing.

3. An office, duty, employment or calling.

4. A particular activity or operation (among several).

5. An official duty.

6. The action of functioning; performance.

We are using the word in its first sense when we say that a guide dog is fulfilling its function by assisting its master to get to work by bus, and in its second sense when we say that the function of a guide dog is to enable its master to get about independently. These meanings of function come close to the sense in which it is used in the *International Classification of Functioning, Disability and Health* (ICF) (World Health Organization 2001). As explained in Chapter 1, this classification system was developed to provide a common language for describing health and health-related states, therefore terms are clearly defined. Body functions are 'the physiological functions of body systems (including psychological functions)' (World Health Organization 2001, p.10), for example, the seeing functions of the eye and the mental functions that govern the speed of the thinking process.

Using the word in its third sense, we might say that the function of keeping communities safe is the responsibility of the police. The concept of function, in this meaning of the word, is closely allied to the idea of duty in many people's minds. For example, if a policeman is found to have accepted a bribe, we might either call this a dereliction of duty or say that he is not fit for the function of policing the community.

We are using the word function in its fourth sense when we say that spreading a mulch of well-rotted manure onto the garden fulfils several different functions, such as saving water in dry weather, keeping the weeds down and providing nutrients for the soil.

The fifth meaning of the word is intended when we say that opening Parliament each year is a function of the Queen. When the word is used in this way, it often carries the connotation of display without substance. The Queen opens Parliament in her capacity as head of state but the real power to govern the country belongs to Parliament, not to the monarch.

The sixth sense of the word comes closer to the second meaning of function in the European conceptual framework. For example, an occupational therapist may talk about assessing a client's level of function in activities of daily living, meaning how well the person performs his everyday tasks. When a doctor says that a person's liver function has been impaired by excessive alcohol consumption, he is using this meaning of the word. In this sense, the word function is sometimes used interchangeably with performance, so we could say that an athlete demonstrates either peak performance or optimum function.

As a verb, function is defined as: fulfil a function; perform a duty or role; act, operate (*Shorter Oxford English Dictionary* 2002). We could say that a person functions well in his role as a care giver, or that someone is not functioning very well today because she has a heavy cold.

How occupational therapists use the term function

The concept of *function* is an important one for occupational therapists, although the word is used in different ways. Katz and Sachs (1991) pointed out that the definitions of occupational therapy concepts, such as occupation, function and doing, vary throughout the literature and that 'usually one or more of them are used to define another concept' (p.137). Unsworth (1993) carried out a literature review to discover how occupational therapists understand function and concluded that 'assessment authors conceptualise function quite differently' (p.288). She went on to say that 'an individual's ability to function is the basis for most occupational therapy practice [but,] in many cases, function is inappropriately defined as being what functional assessments measure' (p.287).

Some examples of the different conceptualizations of function are:

The integrated learning of those adaptive skill components which are needed for successful participation in the social roles expected of the individual in his usual environmental setting. (Mosey 1968, p.428)

An individual's performance of activities, tasks and roles during daily occupations. (Christiansen and Baum 1997, p.5)

An action performed to fulfil an allocated task. (Creek 2003, p.53)

An inability to reach an acceptable or desired level of function is usually called dysfunction. Mosey (1986, p.13) wrote that function and dysfunction are 'considered to be relative to age, cultural background, and the expected environment of the client' so that what would be considered function in one person would be viewed as dysfunction in another. Mosey also suggested that function and dysfunction are on a continuum, meaning that 'there is essentially no break or line of demarcation between that which is considered function and that which is considered dysfunction' (p.13).

How function 1 is understood within the conceptual framework

The first European definition of *function* was constructed from a selection of existing definitions found in the literature that are close in meaning:

••

Function 1 is the underlying physical and psychological components that support occupational performance.

••

This definition is made up of three elements found in existing definitions:

• underlying physical components

• underlying psychological components

• support occupational performance.

To underlie is to form a basis or foundation to something (*Shorter Oxford English Dictionary* 2002). A component, as defined above, is a constituent part of something. So, underlying physical components are the natural activities of the body and underlying psychological components are the natural activities of the mind that together form the foundation for occupational performance. For example, occupational therapists talk about hand function, meaning the different ways in which the hand works, including grasping, releasing, manipulating and so on. Hand function forms part of the foundation for the performance of many occupations.

Function, in this sense of the word, can usually be observed. For example, we can see whether or not someone is able to use their hand to grasp, release, manipulate and so on.

This definition of the term is very close in meaning to the way in which it is used in the ICF (World Health Organization 2001).

How function 2 is understood within the conceptual framework

The second European definition of *function* was also constructed from definitions found in the literature that were close in meaning to each other but different from the meaning of *function 1*:

••

Function 2 is the capacity to use occupational performance components to carry out a task, activity or occupation.

••

This definition is made up of two elements found in existing definitions:

- capacity

- use occupational performance components to carry out a task, activity or occupation.

Capacity is 'an ability...for some specified purpose, activity, or experience' (*Shorter Oxford English Dictionary* 2002). This means that a function is an ability used for the specific purpose of carrying out a task, activity or occupation. For example, we could say that someone who takes a New Year's Day dip in the North Sea has the capacity to tolerate extreme cold.

Occupational performance components, as defined above, are abilities and skills that enable and affect engagement in tasks, activities and occupations. Function, in this second meaning, is the capacity or power to translate abilities and skills into some form of action.

Function, in this sense, cannot be observed directly but can be assumed from the fact that a person is able to carry out a task, activity or occupation. For example, when Robert gets washed and dressed for work in the morning, he is demonstrating that he can function in the area of self-care.

Example 8.2 illustrates the two meanings of function, as used by occupational therapists.

Example 8.2: The two meanings of function

Making a cup of tea is a function in the sense of *function 2*: I require the capacity to use a variety of performance components to carry out this activity. Remembering where I keep the teapot is an example of *function 1*, because registering, storing and retrieving information in the memory are mental functions, as classified in the ICF.

One of the performance components of making a cup of tea is the function of remembering where I keep the teapot. I retain this memory because it is a necessary function for being able to make tea without having to search my kitchen for the pot. There are several different memory functions involved in finding the teapot, including remembering that I am looking for it, remembering what the pot looks like, remembering that I keep it in a kitchen cupboard, remembering which cupboard, remembering how to open the door and remembering how to hold the teapot.

Some people have more effective function than others in particular activities. For example, a professional tennis player is likely to have more effective function in demanding physical activities than a computer programmer. Most people's level of function varies at different times, depending on internal and external circumstances: for example, a marathon runner expects his level of function to improve when he is in training for a race.

ABILITY

This section discusses the common usage of the term *ability*, then the ways in which it is used by occupational therapists and, finally, the European definition.

What ability means in common usage

Ability is a concept commonly used in many social settings, such as education, work, sport and the arts. The *Shorter Oxford English Dictionary* (2002) gives several meanings of the word, including legal competency (to act) and pecuniary power, neither of which is relevant in this context. Six definitions are relevant to this chapter:

1. Suitable or sufficient power.

2. Capacity (to do something).

3. Bodily power.

4. Mental power.

5. A special power of the mind, a faculty.

6. Talent, cleverness.

We are using the word in its first sense when we say that a girl has the ability to become a first class tennis player, or that one boxer has the ability to beat another one.

In the second meaning of the word, we might say that someone has a remarkable ability to play chess, or that a footballer always plays to the best of his ability. In this sense, ability usually refers to a particular type of activity, so the person with a remarkable ability to play chess may not have a similar ability to play football. This meaning of the word is close to the meaning given in the European conceptual framework.

Ability can refer to bodily power, for example, we could say that long distance runners have the ability to maintain speed and stamina over great distances. It can also refer to mental power, as when we say that someone has limited creative ability.

In the fifth sense, ability means being competent in a particular type of action. For example, some people with autism have special mathematical or artistic ability, although their ability in other areas may be limited. The neurologist, Oliver Sacks (1986), described a young man with severe learning disability and autism who had the ability to make precise and accurate drawings from life or from memory.

Leonardo da Vinci was said to have the ability to draw a perfect circle freehand: this is using the word in its sixth sense.

Ability is a word usually employed to describe positive attributes; those capacities and powers that are valued in society, such as strength and cleverness. However, we could also say that a person has the ability to do something bad or unacceptable, such as the ability to ignore a child in distress or the ability to inflict cruelty on animals.

The ICF (World Health Organization 2001) describes disability in terms of capacity limitation rather than ability limitation.

How occupational therapists use the term ability

The concept of *ability* is less often found in the occupational therapy literature than the related concepts of *skill* and *function*. Mosey (1968) defined skills in terms of abilities: for example, perceptual-motor skill is made up of six abilities, including 'the ability to recognize body parts and their relationship to one another' (p.426) and 'the ability to perform ordinary activities of daily living and specific motor tasks' (p.427).

Christiansen and Baum (1997) observed that the terms *ability* and *skill* are often used interchangeably by occupational therapists but that 'it is useful to view them as distinct concepts' (p.56). They defined ability as a general trait that is a product of genetic make-up and learning, and said that abilities are brought forth when someone learns a new task. Examples of abilities are spatial orientation, selective attention, dynamic strength and reaction time. Impairment of ability is called functional limitation.

The South African occupational therapist, Vona du Toit (1991), developed a model for occupational therapy practice called the model of creative ability. She defined *creative ability* as:

> Manifested in [the individual's] creation of a tangible or intangible product. The quality of his action (Doing) reflects the quality of the volitional component of his 'Being'. The level of his 'Doing' is characterised by the level of his ability to form relational contacts with materials, people and situations, by the measure of his anxiety control,

by his manifestation of originative ability and by the quality of his preparedness to actualise himself through exercising effort in action which makes maximal demands on his potential. (du Toit 1991, p.39)

Forsyth and Kielhofner (2006) described ability as performance capacity, such as range of motion, strength or cognition, contrasting it with skills, which are the discrete actions seen during occupational performance.

How ability is understood within the conceptual framework

The European definition of *ability* was constructed from existing definitions found in the literature:

> An *ability* is a personal characteristic that supports occupational performance.

This definition was constructed from two elements found in existing definitions:

- a personal characteristic

- supports occupational performance.

A personal characteristic is 'a distinguishing trait, peculiarity, or quality' (*Shorter Oxford English Dictionary* 2002) that belongs to the person as an individual, rather than as a member of a group. For example, Judith is a good listener; this is a personal characteristic.

Ability is an occupational performance component, as described in an earlier section. Ability enables and affects the performance of tasks, activities and occupations. In her job as a Mental Health Act Commissioner, Judith is expected to listen carefully and respectfully to the stories of detained patients: having the capacity to pay careful attention when someone is speaking (*ability*) supports her performance in this job.

SKILL

The concept of *skill* is frequently found in the occupational therapy literature, illustrating how important it is to both theory and practice. This section begins with a discussion of what *skill* means in common usage and then explores some of the ways in which the term has been used by occupational therapists. It finishes with an explanation of how *skill* is defined in the European conceptual framework.

What skill means in common usage

The *Shorter Oxford English Dictionary* (2002) gives several meanings of the word *skill*, including: reasonableness, discrimination, discretion and justice, none of which is relevant in this context. Three definitions are relevant to this chapter:

1. Ability to do something (esp. manual or physical) well.

2. Proficiency, expertness, dexterity.

3. An ability to do something, acquired through practice or learning.

We are using the word in its first meaning when we say that a gambler has a great deal of skill at cards, or that a magician has the skill to create illusions for his audience. Although the dictionary states that this type of skill is usually manual or physical, other abilities may be involved in demonstrating the skill, such as cognitive or interpersonal abilities.

In the second sense of the word, we might say that it takes a great deal of skill to grow pineapples in the UK, or that a speech writer must have skill with words.

The third definition of skill comes very close to the meaning given to the term in the European conceptual framework. We are using it in this sense when we talk about children learning the skill of reading or the skill of mental arithmetic.

How occupational therapists use the term skill

The term *skill* is much more widely used by occupational therapists than the related term, *ability*, but there is little agreement on how to define it. For example, an early model for occupational therapy practice, recapitulation of ontogenesis, was based on the idea that: 'comfortable and productive existence requires the capacity to adapt...adaptation requires the learning of specific patterns of behavior [and] these behavioral patterns are referred to...as "adaptive skills"' (Mosey 1968, p.426). The model describes seven adaptive skills, which are learned in parallel as the child develops: perceptual-motor, cognitive, drive-object, dyadic interaction, primary group interaction, self-identity and sexual identity interaction skills.

Reed and Sanderson (1992, p.91) offered a similar definition of skills: 'learned behaviors acquired by practice and experience'. They identified three types of skill: sensorimotor, cognitive and psychosocial skills.

Hagedorn (1995, p.61) offered an alternative perspective on skills, suggesting that they are 'both innate potentials and the transference of those potentials into effective practice'. This definition comes close to the meaning of skill within the European conceptual framework.

Christiansen and Baum (1997, p.57) offered a third understanding of skill: 'the level of proficiency in a specific task'. They suggested that skills are underpinned by 'various underlying general abilities' (p.57), for example, the skill of driving a car is determined by such abilities as reaction time, perceptual speed, peripheral vision and motor control.

Hagedorn (2000) made a further attempt to clarify the meaning of skill, giving it a similar meaning to that proposed by Christiansen and Baum and saying that the word 'describes *how* a thing is done, not *the thing being done*' (p.31). This means that there are levels of skill and that an action can be performed well or badly. For example, driving is a skill but not everyone drives well.

Two Danish occupational therapists, Fortmeier and Thanning (2002), described an approach to occupational therapy practice based on Russian activity theory, in which skills are a prerequisite for activity and are developed through activity. Skills and needs create the motives for action, action develops new skills and needs which, in turn, lead to further action.

The UK definition of occupational therapy as a complex intervention defined a skill as 'a specific ability or integrated set of abilities (e.g. motor, sensory, cognitive or perceptual) which evolve with practice' (Creek 2003, p.59). During an intervention, the occupational therapist shifts her focus of attention from occupation, to activity, to task, to skill and back again, in order to ensure that skill development is having a positive impact on task, activity and occupational performance.

Forsyth and Kielhofner (2006) defined a skill as a discrete, purposeful action and said that sequences of these actions make up occupational performance. This definition is similar to the concept of *task*, as defined in Chapter 4. Forsyth and Kielhofner identified three types of skills: motor; process, and communication and interaction skills.

A further definition of skill was offered by Roberts (2008, p.360): 'something we know how to do and feel comfortable with when putting it into action'. Roberts linked the concept of *skill* to two of the other concepts explored in this chapter, *occupational performance component* and *ability*. She said that a skill is a performance component that evolves with practice, and that skills are dependent on abilities. For example, driving is a skill that improves with practice and that is dependent on such abilities as visual-spatial perception and range of motion.

The word competence is sometimes used interchangeably with skill but Hagedorn (2000, p.55) argued that they are 'not truly interchangeable'. Mastering a set of skills brings proficiency in a situation or task, while competence refers to the degree of proficiency. For example, being able to read numbers and tell the time are necessary skills for becoming proficient in the use of public transport but some people are better able than others to find their way around the public transport system, that is, they are more competent.

Occupational therapists are not just concerned with the skills of their clients but have also studied their own professional skills. For example, a paper published in 1989 identified four types of professional skill: required clinical practices and procedures; core professional skills; common professional skills, and special skills acquired through individual interest (Joice and Coia 1989).

The study of occupational therapy as a complex intervention (Creek 2003) found that occupational therapists have a range of core skills and an additional range of thinking skills. Core professional skills are:

- collaboration with the client

- assessment of function

- enablement

- problem-solving

- using activity as a therapeutic tool

- group work

- environmental adaptation.

The thinking skills of the occupational therapist are:

- clinical reasoning, including scientific, narrative, interactive, conditional, pragmatic and ethical reasoning

- reflection.

How skill is understood within the conceptual framework

The European definition of *skill* was constructed from definitions found in the literature:

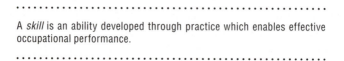

A *skill* is an ability developed through practice which enables effective occupational performance.

This definition is made up of three elements found in existing definitions:

- an ability

- developed through practice

- enables effective occupational performance.

An ability, as defined above, is a personal characteristic that supports occupational performance. We could say that Roger has the ability to hold his breath under water for up to a minute.

In order to be seen as a skill, an ability has to be developed through practice. For example, Roger practised holding his breath under water until he could manage it for more than two minutes: he developed the skill of holding his breath under water.

A skill enables effective occupational performance. Someone could have an ability, developed through practice, but it would not count as a skill unless he could use it to perform effectively. For example, Roger wants to be able to hold his breath under water so that he can dive without oxygen. However, he is only able to hold his breath while floating, not while swimming, so this ability has not yet developed into the skill that he is aiming for.

RELATIONSHIPS BETWEEN TERMS REPRESENTING PERSONAL REQUISITES FOR ACTION

The range of tasks, activities and occupations that a person is able to undertake is determined by his physical and psychological components (*function 1*), his occupational performance components (*abilities* and *skills*) and his capacity to use those components to carry out a task, activity or occupation (*function 2*). The more functions a person has, and the more occupational performance components he is able to use, the wider will be the range of occupations available to him.

Each person is born with an array of potentials, such as the potential to learn to walk. These potentials are dependent on his functions, such as the mobility and stability of his joints and the tone of his muscles (*function 1*). As the child grows, he develops certain abilities, such as the ability to start walking at a certain age. With practice, he learns skills, such as being able to walk independently, to adjust his pace and to walk on rough surfaces.

Shifting perspectives

Relationships between concepts in the cluster of personal requisites for action are not fixed but change depending on the context and on the perspective of the person engaging in occupational performance. For example, a performance component might be perceived as an ability or a skill, as shown in Example 8.3.

Example 8.3: Ability or skill?

An *ability* is a personal characteristic that supports occupational performance, such as Herman's mathematical ability, which supports him in his work as a tax accountant. A *skill* is an ability developed through practice which enables effective occupational performance, such as Herman's skill in completing tax returns, which has been honed through years of practice, enabling him to be good at his job.

However, Herman's mathematical ability has been improved and maintained with practice, and he is an effective tax accountant, so it could be said that his numerical dexterity is a skill rather than an ability. Conversely, most academic mathematicians are better at manipulating numbers than Herman, so his occupational performance in this area could be improved. Whether an element of performance is seen as a skill or an ability shifts and changes depending on the perspective from which it is viewed.

The physical and psychological components that support performance (*function 1*) can only be observed when they are used to carry out a task, activity or occupation (*function 2*). For example, the ICF describes three emotional functions: appropriateness of emotion, regulation of emotion and range of emotion (World Health Organization 2001). The person experiencing emotion might be aware of these three functions but an observer would be able to assess them only through their expression in a real-life situation, as shown in Example 8.4.

Example 8.4: Observing emotional functions

When Derek was referred to the community occupational therapist, he had a 15-year history of severe depression, which had caused him to drop out of university in his second year. During their first meeting, the therapist observed that Derek looked depressed and his facial expression was immobile. He used the same flat tone of voice when talking about painful life events, such as his girlfriend leaving him, and about happy events, such as going to a rock concert with friends.

As the therapist got to know Derek, her first impression was confirmed that he experienced a limited range of emotions; in particular, he did not experience strong feelings such as pleasure, excitement, anticipation or anger. This meant that he was often unable to feel emotions that were appropriate to the occasion. When the therapist shared her observations with Derek, he agreed with her and said that he would like to learn how to experience and express a wider range of emotions. This became one of the main goals of the occupational therapy intervention.

SUMMARY

This chapter explored the four terms used by occupational therapists to refer to personal requisites for action: *occupational performance components, function, skill* and *ability*. The first term is not used by the general public but the common meaning of the other three words was explored. The ways that all four terms are used in the occupational therapy literature were discussed. The European definitions of the terms were given, with explanations of how the definitions were constructed and what they mean. The word *function* has been given two definitions, reflecting the two different meanings it has for occupational therapists. The final part of the chapter considered the relationships between the four terms, highlighting the dynamic nature of those relationships.

The next chapter looks at the second cluster of terms in the internal world of the performer: the energy source for action.

REFERENCES

Canadian Association of Occupational Therapists, Health Canada (1993) *Occupational Therapy Guidelines for Client-centred Mental Health Practice.* Toronto: CAOT Publications ACE.

Chapparo, C. and Ranka, J. (2005) 'Theoretical contexts.' In G. Whiteford and V. Wright-St Clair (eds) *Occupation in Practice and Context.* Sydney: Elsevier Churchill Livingstone.

Christiansen, C. and Baum, C. (1997) 'Person-environment Occupational Performance: a conceptual model for practice.' In C. Christiansen and C. Baum (eds) *Occupational Therapy: Enabling Function and Well-being, Second Edition.* Thorofare, NJ: Slack.

Creek, J. (1998) 'Purposeful activity.' In J. Creek (ed.) *Occupational Therapy: New Perspectives.* London: Whurr.

Creek, J. (2003) *Occupational Therapy Defined as a Complex Intervention.* London: College of Occupational Therapists.

Cronin-Davis, J., Lang, A. and Molineux, M. (2004) 'Occupational science: the forensic challenge.' In M. Molineux (ed.) *Occupation for Occupational Therapists.* Oxford: Blackwell.

Department of National Health and Welfare & Canadian Association of Occupational Therapists (1983) *Guidelines for the Client-centred Practice of Occupational Therapy.* (H39-33/1983E.) Ottawa: Department of National Health and Welfare.

du Toit, V. (1991) *Patient Volition and Action in Occupational Therapy, Second Edition.* Hillbrow: Vona & Marie du Toit Foundation.

Forsyth, K. and Kielhofner, G. (2006) 'The Model of Human Occupation: integrating theory into practice and practice into theory.' In E.A.S. Duncan (ed.) *Foundations for Practice in Occupational Therapy, Fourth Edition.* Edinburgh: Elsevier Churchill Livingstone.

Fortmeier, S. and Thanning, G. (2002) *From the Patient's Point of View: An Activity Theory Approach to Occupational Therapy.* Copenhagen: Ergoterapeutforeningen.

Hagedorn, R. (1995) *Occupational Therapy: Perspectives and Processes.* Edinburgh: Churchill Livingstone.

Hagedorn, R. (2000) *Tools for Practice in Occupational Therapy: A Structured Approach to Core Skills and Processes.* Edinburgh: Churchill Livingstone.

Joice, A. and Coia, D. (1989) 'A discussion of the skills of the occupational therapist working within a multidisciplinary team.' *British Journal of Occupational Therapy 52,* 12, 466–468.

Katz, N. and Sachs, D. (1991) 'Meaning ascribed to major professional concepts: a comparison of occupational therapy students and practitioners in the United States and Israel.' *American Journal of Occupational Therapy 45,* 2, 137–145.

Molineux, M. (2004) 'Occupation in occupational therapy: a labour in vain?' In M. Molineux (ed.) *Occupation for Occupational Therapists.* Oxford: Blackwell.

Mosey, A.C. (1968) 'Recapitulation of ontogenesis: a theory for practice of occupational therapy.' *American Journal of Occupational Therapy 22,* 5, 426–438.

Mosey, A.C. (1986) *Psychosocial Components of Occupational Therapy.* New York: Raven Press.

Reed, K.L. and Sanderson, S.N. (1992) *Concepts of Occupational Therapy, Third Edition.* Baltimore, MD: Williams and Wilkins.

Roberts, M. (2008) 'Life skills.' In J. Creek and L. Lougher (eds) *Occupational Therapy and Mental Health, Fourth Edition.* Edinburgh: Churchill Livingstone Elsevier.

Sacks, O. (1986) *The Man Who Mistook his Wife for a Hat.* London: Picador.

Shorter Oxford English Dictionary, Fifth Edition (2002). Oxford: Oxford University Press.

Sumsion, T. and Blank, A. (2006) 'The Canadian Model of Occupational Performance.' In E.A.S. Duncan (ed.) *Foundations for Practice in Occupational Therapy, Fourth Edition.* Edinburgh: Elsevier Churchill Livingstone.

Unsworth, C. (1993) 'The concept of function.' *British Journal of Occupational Therapy 56,* 8, 287–292.

Wilby, H.J. (2007) 'The importance of maintaining a focus on performance components in occupational therapy practice.' *British Journal of Occupational Therapy 70,* 3, 129–132.

World Health Organization (2001) *ICF: International Classification of Functioning, Disability and Health.* Geneva: World Health Organization.

CHAPTER 9

ENERGY SOURCE FOR ACTION

INTRODUCTION

The purpose of this chapter, together with the last chapter, is to explore the internal world of the performer, where the energy and other personal requisites for action are located. The personal components of occupational performance were discussed in Chapter 8. In this chapter we will be exploring three terms that, together, describe where the energy for action comes from and how it is directed into one activity rather than another. These terms are *motivation, volition* and *engagement*.

'The occupational therapist believes that the drive to act is a basic human need' (Creek 2003, p.28). People are naturally active beings, who do not need to be given reasons to engage in activity, but different people choose to do different things and their choices can be made for many reasons. Choices are always limited, by internal conditions or external circumstances. All these issues will be discussed in this chapter.

MOTIVATION

The concept of *motivation* is central to occupational therapy practice. Since the profession was founded at the beginning of the twentieth century, occupational therapists have been concerned with their clients' motivation to engage in therapeutic activities and more recently, as interventions have moved towards community settings, their motivation to participate in life situations.

The theories of motivation used by occupational therapists are drawn mainly from the discipline of psychology, although some theorists have attempted to embed them within occupational therapy approaches and models (for example, du Toit 1991; Mosey 1986; Reilly 1974).

What motivation means in common usage

The *Shorter Oxford English Dictionary* (2002) states that the noun *motivation* comes from the verbs *motive* and *motivate*, which mean:

1. Supply or be a motive for (an action); provide (a person etc.) with a motive or incentive (to do); stimulate the interest of (a person) in an activity.

2. Serve as a reason for, justify (a decision etc.).

A *motive* (noun) is: a factor or circumstance inducing a person to act in a certain way; an emotion, reason, goal, etc. influencing or tending to influence a person's volition.

Four definitions of *motivation* are given in the *Shorter Oxford English Dictionary*:

1. The action or act of motivating something or someone.

2. The (conscious or unconscious) stimulus, incentive, motives, etc., for action towards a goal, esp. as resulting from psychological or social factors; the factors giving purpose or direction to behaviour.

3. The state or condition of being motivated; the degree to which a person is motivated; enthusiasm, drive.

4. (A) manner or means of movement.

In the first sense of the word, we might say that a lecturer provides the motivation for his students to arrive on time for lectures by always beginning with a surprise, such as a joke or an unexpected demonstration. This use of the word suggests that motivation is an interaction between the external world (the lecturer's strategy for getting students to arrive on time) and the internal world of the performer (the student's response to the lecturer's strategy).

The second and third meanings of motivation are close to the way in which the term is used in the European conceptual framework. The second definition refers to the extrinsic factors that move a person to act (stimulus, incentive, motives). These motivating factors may be external (social), such as the possibility of promotion at work, or internal (psychological), such as the desire to win. The individual may know why she wants to act in a particular way (conscious motive) or be aware of the urge to act but not know where her motivation comes from (unconscious motive). This definition also suggests that motivating factors influence a person to act in a particular way (giving purpose or direction). So, when using the word in this sense, we might say that a woman's motivation to lose weight is the desire to wear a size 12 dress for her wedding.

In its third meaning, motivation refers to the experience of the performer; the feeling that she has when doing something. We are using the term in this sense when we say that a climber feels an overwhelming motivation to reach the summit of Everest, or that an actor's motivation to perform well is enhanced by knowing that a famous critic is in the audience.

Motivation is not often used in its fourth sense; the words motion or locomotion are more common. This meaning of the word is not relevant to this chapter.

The concept of motivation is of particular interest in the fields of work and education. Managers want to find the best ways to keep their workers motivated and teachers are keen to promote their pupils' enthusiasm for learning. For example, the American sociologist, Sennett (2008), in his exploration of the nature of craftsmanship, compared the effectiveness of individual competition versus group cooperation in motivating people to work well. He also suggested that everyone has the potential to become a good craftsman but 'it is the motivation and aspiration for quality that takes people along different paths in their lives' (ibid., p.241).

The *International Classification of Functioning, Disability and Health* (ICF) (World Health Organization 2001) includes a category for energy and drive functions, one of which is motivation.

Motivation has been extensively studied by psychologists, as an intrinsic aspect of human behaviour: 'The concept of motivation is central in our attempt to understand behavior and its causes' (Smith 1993, p.367). There are numerous psychological perspectives and theories of motivation, which can be found in any standard psychology textbook.

One theory of motivation that is important to occupational therapists is the distinction between intrinsic and extrinsic motivation. Intrinsic motivation is a basic drive to act; it pushes us to act for the pleasure of being active. Extrinsic motivation is the drive to meet needs, attain goals, win rewards or avoid punishment. Extrinsic motivators may be internal, such as a feeling of hunger, or external, such as the promise of a pay rise. Theories of intrinsic and extrinsic motivation will be discussed later in this chapter.

How occupational therapists use the term motivation

As stated in the introduction to this section, occupational therapists are fully aware of the importance of motivation in their clients. However, their attention has been focused mainly on intrinsic motivation.

> Despite the fact that numerous theories of motivation exist, not all are relevant to the practice of occupational therapy. Only theories of intrinsic motivation recognize that humans engage in activity for its own sake, and not for the benefit of extrinsic rewards or to fulfill unconscious needs. (Doble 1988, p.75)

Dr Elizabeth Casson, who founded the first school of occupational therapy in the UK, suggested that curiosity is one of the most powerful intrinsic motivators and that 'the well-trained occupational therapist uses this active motive in her patients continually' (Casson 1955, p.99). She also saw achievement as a key factor in motivating people to engage in activity. Referring to the treatment of children in an orthopaedic hospital, she wrote:

> Following on the instinct of curiosity comes the desire to achieve. Every child loves to make something that he has made himself, and the pleasure is even greater if he can send something home that he has made and that earns the praise of his family. (Casson 1955, p.99)

This theory of intrinsic motivation was further developed by Mary Reilly, at the University of Southern California. She wrote a book about the role of play in children's learning, in which she suggested that:

> Play behavior we know is permeated by the exploratory drive of curiosity... The readiness state of curiosity, it is speculated, has three hierarchical stages, namely exploratory, competency, and achievement. These progressive stages are hypothesized as expressing a higher level of excitement and requiring a corresponding need for more control. While curiosity may be the basic motivation driving the system, the three

derivative areas of exploration, competency, and achievement appear to function in a relatively autonomous way. (Reilly 1974, pp.145–146)

In 1977, one of Reilly's colleagues, Janice Burke, reviewed existing psychological theories of motivation and judged that they were all inadequate for occupational therapists. She put forward a theory based on the concept of personal causation, which is: 'the initiation by the individual of behavior intended to produce a change in his environment' (de Charms 1968, cited by Burke 1977, p.256). Personal causation incorporates four factors that the occupational therapist should consider in order to promote motivated behaviour in patients.

> The four perspectives described to assess the capacity for motivation and to guide the clinical promotion of it when it fails to emerge or is disrupted by disease are: expectancies of success or failure, internal versus external orientation, belief in skill, and a sense of efficacy. (Burke 1977, p.258)

Much of Burke's work on intrinsic motivation became subsumed into later theories of volition, leading to a period of confusion between the two concepts. This will be explored further in the section on how occupational therapists use the term *volition*.

Christiansen and Baum (1997) developed a person-environment-occupational performance model for occupational therapy practice, in which personal causation was described as one of a number of cognitive theories of motivation. Cognitive theories 'explain that people motivate themselves by formulating goals, and planning and regulating their actions to attain them' (*ibid.*, p.50). Key features of motivation are:

- internality – 'the extent to which people feel that their actions can influence the environment' (*ibid.*, p.51)

- self-efficacy – 'a person's feelings of competence' (p.51)

- personality – 'the interests, values and attitudes of an individual that influence their attention, behavior, and interpretation of new events' (*ibid.*, p.51)

- values – 'beliefs and interpretive sentiments that influence choice, conduct and meaning in daily life' (*ibid.*, p.52)

- meaning – 'our overall interpretations of life events' (*ibid.*, p.53)

- spiritual meaning – 'an individual's sense of self and his or her beliefs about power, control and meaning in life' (*ibid.*, p.54).

Vona du Toit, a South African occupational therapist, defined motivation as 'a drive towards action' (1991, p.47). She observed that this drive is not constant but varies between individuals and within the same individual at different times. Du Toit developed a theory of human activity which identifies six levels of motivation from tone, the lowest, to competitive contribution, the highest.

Creek (2007) suggested that motivation is only one of the factors that contribute to an individual's energy for engaging in activity; the other key factors being volition and autonomy. The concept of *autonomy* was explored in Chapter 7 and *volition* is discussed later in this chapter.

How motivation is understood within the conceptual framework

The European definition of *motivation* was constructed from definitions of the term found in the literature:

. . . .

Motivation is a drive that directs a person's actions towards meeting needs.

. . . .

This definition was constructed from three elements found in existing definitions of motivation:

- a drive

- directs a person's actions

- towards meeting needs.

A drive is 'an inner urge to satisfy some basic need or motivation' (*Shorter Oxford English Dictionary* 2002). An example of a drive is the urge to eat, which is an expression of the basic need for food and is experienced as hunger.

Motivation is not a generalized drive to act but is directed towards actions that will satisfy a particular urge. So, when a person is hungry, he has the specific urge to eat and not to play tennis. When he is tired, he has the urge to sleep, not to do a crossword puzzle.

People have the capacity to act in order to meet their needs, or to work towards meeting their needs. These may be immediate needs, such as the need to drink when you are thirsty, or long-term needs, such as the need to gain a qualification in order to earn a living. As children grow up they develop, to a greater or lesser extent, the ability to defer immediate gratification of many of their needs in order to achieve long-term goals. For example, a student may work late to finish an essay, despite being tired and needing to go to sleep.

As described in the introduction, human beings have a basic need to be active, 'to act for the enjoyment of exercising one's capacities, for learning and for taking pleasure in activity' (Creek 2007, p.130). This drive is what we call intrinsic motivation.

VOLITION

The concept of *volition* was not widely used by occupational therapists before the 1980s; instead, they wrote about motivation and about choice. In 1980, four papers were published in the *American Journal of Occupational Therapy*, describing a new model for practice in which volition was a central concept (Kielhofner 1980a, 1980b; Kielhofner and Burke 1980; Kielhofner, Burke and Igi 1980). There followed a period of confusion in which occupational therapists conflated the concepts of motivation and volition, using the latter to mean both drive and choice. These issues are discussed in this section.

What volition means in common usage

The *Shorter Oxford English Dictionary* (2002) gives three definitions of *volition*:

1. An act of willing or resolving something; a decision or choice made after due consideration or deliberation.

2. The action of consciously willing or resolving something; the making of a definite choice or decision regarding a course of action; exercise of the will.

3. The power or faculty of willing; will-power.

An example of using volition in the sense of the first definition would be to say that a person exercised his volition when deciding to give up a career in medicine and retrain to be an architect.

In the second sense of the word, we might talk about a person leaving his job of his own volition, meaning that he freely chose to leave.

In the third sense, we could say that a woman who wants to give up smoking but is unable to do so lacks volition, meaning that she does not have the will-power to stop.

Having the capacity to exercise volition, or to make one's own decisions, is a highly valued quality in societies that also value individualism and independence. To be weak-willed, or deficient in volition, may be seen as a moral weakness. For example, fat people are sometimes derided for not having the will-power to eat less or to eat less fattening food, or a compulsive gambler is seen as immoral for spending his money on betting instead of paying the bills.

In psychiatry, reduced volition is perceived as a negative symptom of chronic schizophrenia: 'The most striking feature is diminished volition, that is a lack of drive and initiative. Left to himself, the patient may be inactive for long periods, or may engage in aimless and repeated activity' (Gelder, Gath and Mayou 1989 p.272).

How occupational therapists use the term volition

As described in the introduction to this section, the term *volition* was not widely used in the occupational therapy literature until 1980, when it was introduced in a model for practice by two American occupational therapists: *A Model of Human Occupation*. This model used general systems theory as an organizing framework and described a person as an open system consisting of three internal sub-systems: volition, habituation and performance. The volition sub-system was described as 'the urge that motivates occupation' (Kielhofner and Burke 1980, p.575), a definition that is close in meaning to the European definition of *motivation*.

Following the publication of this paper, and subsequent publications on the model, occupational therapists appeared to become confused about the nature of motivation and volition, treating them as though they were the same concept. For example, a paper published in 1994 described the volition sub-system of the model of human occupation as both a 'conceptualization of motivation' and a concept that explained 'choices for action' (Helfrich, Kielhofner and Mattingly 1994, p.313).

Du Toit (1991) also developed a model for practice, the model of creative ability, in which the concepts of volition and motivation are conflated. Creative ability is 'the way in which people realize, define and extend themselves by expressing their potential through creative action'

(Creek 2008, p.338). One component of creative ability is 'an inner motivation of drive towards action', which is called volition (du Toit 1991,
p.47).

A comprehensive definition of occupational therapy, published by the
UK College of Occupational Therapists, made a distinction between the
concepts of motivation and volition, taking definitions of the two terms
from the *Oxford English Dictionary* (Creek 2003):

- Motivation is 'the conscious or unconscious stimulus, incentive,
  motives etc. for action towards a goal' (*ibid.*, p.55).

- Volition is 'exercise of the will; the mental action of consciously
  willing or resolving something, or making a choice or decision
  regarding a course of action' (*ibid.*, p.61).

In a later publication, Creek (2007) further clarified the difference between motivation and volition, describing motivation as 'the drive to
act' (p.129) and volition as 'the skill of being able to make autonomous
choices and decisions about what action to take' (p.134).

How volition is understood within the conceptual framework

The European definition of *volition* was constructed from definitions of
the term found in the literature:

....

Volition is the ability to choose to do or continue to do something, together
with an awareness that the performance of the activity is voluntary.

....

This definition was constructed from four elements found in existing
definitions of *volition*:

- ability

- to choose to do something

- to choose to continue to do something

- together with an awareness that the performance of the activity
  is voluntary.

An ability is a personal characteristic that supports occupational performance, as discussed in Chapter 8. So, we might say that someone
has the ability to play the violin, meaning that he has the necessary

qualities to choose, organize and carry out that activity as part of one of his occupations.

To choose to do something is to exercise free will in selecting a course of action and initiating that action. For example, Jane decides to have a weekend in Edinburgh so she selects a weekend when she has no other commitments and books train tickets and a hotel room.

To choose to continue to do something means not stopping a task or activity when one has the opportunity to do so. For example, Peter and Margaret go for a walk along a section of a long distance footpath. There are several points at which they could leave the path and take a bus home, but the weather is fine so they decide to continue walking until it starts to get dark.

To be aware that the performance of an activity is voluntary means knowing that one is exercising free will, that one does not have to do the activity or that one can stop doing it. For example, Debbie could afford to pay for residential care for her elderly mother but chooses to look after her at home, even though it is hard work. She acknowledges that this is her own choice.

ENGAGEMENT

The concept of *engagement* has been familiar to occupational therapists since the foundation of the profession, although it went out of fashion for some years. Two American occupational therapists, Hooper and Wood (2002), proposed that occupational therapy has developed with two incompatible epistemologies, pragmatism and structuralism, and that one or other is in the ascendant at any particular time. The concept of engagement would seem to fit comfortably within a pragmatist world view and it is now coming back into vogue, along with other pragmatic approaches to practice such as client-centred practice and narrative reasoning.

In common usage, engagement has a more limited meaning than that given to it by occupational therapists, as explained in this section.

What engagement means in common usage

According to the *Shorter Oxford English Dictionary* (2002), the word *engagement* has seven meanings, including: a legal or moral obligation; a tie or attachment, and an encounter between parties at war. The meaning that is most relevant in this context is: 'a piece of business requiring a person's attention or presence; *esp.* a paid appointment, a job'.

This is a narrow definition of engagement when compared with the meaning it has for occupational therapists, as discussed below. In the sense of this definition, we might say that a person cannot have lunch with her friend today because she has a prior engagement, or we could say that a comedian has an engagement to perform in a club for a week.

The verb *to engage* has a wide range of meanings, several of which are of relevance to occupational therapists:

1. Urge, persuade, induce.

2. Fascinate, charm.

3. Involve, entangle.

4. Enter upon or occupy oneself in an activity, interest etc.

5. Keep occupied or busy, provide occupation for (a person, a person's thoughts, etc.).

6. Attract and hold fast (a person's attention, interest, etc.).

The first sense of the word is being used when an entrepreneur tries to engage a financier to invest in his business. In the second sense, we might say that someone has an engaging manner, meaning that he is good company. The third sense of engage is more likely to be found in its negative form: to disengage, for example a man complains that he is finding it difficult to disengage from a relationship he no longer finds rewarding.

The fourth and fifth meanings of the word are closest to the way in which engagement is used in the European conceptual framework. In the fourth sense, we might talk about someone engaging in a neighbourhood renewal project, or engaging in wrongdoing. We are using the word in the fifth sense when we say that someone is engaged in identifying all the birds that visit her garden over the course of a year. In the final sense of the word, we might talk about trying to engage someone's attention, meaning that we want them to take an interest in what we are saying or doing.

Several other words are sometimes used in a similar sense to the way that occupational therapists use *engagement*, such as flow and mindfulness. These are discussed in more detail in the next section.

How occupational therapists use the term engagement

As stated in the introduction to this section, the concept of *engagement* has been central to occupational therapy since the profession was founded. In an article from 1933, Haworth wrote that patients with both physical and mental health conditions can benefit from activities that engage their attention, in the sense of interesting them. For example, whereas people with arthritis 'tend to resist passive movements which cause them pain, when interested in some special form of work, they use their hands or limbs willingly and tend to forget the pain' (Haworth 1933, p.171). In the field of mental health, 'the purpose of the occupation is to engage the patient's mind so that while she is at work the sense of depression, or the delusions from which she suffers, or the hallucinations which distress her when her attention is not otherwise held, are driven out' (*ibid.*, p.173).

An American physician, Engelhardt, in a paper written in 1977, argued that occupational therapy 'appeals to broad and basic human values of activity and engagement in reality' (Engelhardt 1977, p.670). He referred to the roots of occupational therapy in moral treatment:

> The point of a comparison between moral treatment and occupational therapy is a common model of health or disease, one with a focus on human engagement in tasks. After all, the derivation of occupation is from *occupatio*, a seizing, a taking possession. It is interesting that *occupatio*, in fact, had by transference two further meanings – employment and anticipation – the elements of engagement in reality and of the structuring of time that occupational therapy came to stress. (Engelhardt 1977, p.668)

A study of the clinical reasoning of occupational therapists, carried out in the United States in the 1990s, found that when occupational therapists talk about 'engagement in activity' they are expressing both an idea and a value: 'The idea is that engagement is an involvement and a sense of connection with the activity, an investment in the activity; the value is that it is important to be engaged in what one does' (Fleming 1994, p.97).

Occupational scientists have also taken an interest in the concept of engagement. For example, Carlson (1996, p.145), in a paper on the self-perpetuating property of occupations, coined the phrase occupational perseverance to refer to 'prolonged engagement in an occupation that is directly or indirectly related to prior engagement with the occupation in question'.

A study investigating the occupations of five patients detained in two forensic medium secure units focused on participants' experience of occupational engagement (Stewart and Craik 2007). The concept of engagement was not defined but various terms were used to explain it, including meaning, structure, enjoyment, feeling competent, choice, autonomy and motivation.

Engagement has been described as 'an important process in working with people with severe and enduring mental health problems, whether this be the first contact or continuing engagement' (Hughes 2008, p.418). In this context, engagement refers both to the quality of the client's involvement with activity and of his relationship with the therapist.

In recent years, some occupational therapy authors have borrowed terms from other fields to describe the quality of the client's involvement in activity, rather than using engagement. A paper on boredom described it as 'a feeling of frustration and restlessness, with time spent trying to find something to do that would engage them' (Martin 2009, p.41). Yet, despite this association of boredom with lack of engagement, the author recommended that 'the solution...for dealing with boredom is learning how to be more mindful' (p.41). Mindfulness is described as a form of meditation in which the individual deliberately pays attention to the experience of the present moment, a different concept from engagement, which occupational therapists describe as involvement rather than attention.

Another word that occupational therapists sometimes use to refer to people's experience of activity is flow, which is 'a psychological state that occurs when a person is so involved in an occupation that he or she forgets everything except what he or she is doing and the perception of time is altered' (Timmons and MacDonald 2008, p.87). For example, a phenomenological study of ceramics as a creative leisure activity elicited positive comments from participants about their involvement in the activity, such as 'you become lost in the work and time passes very quickly' (*ibid.*, p.90). The authors chose to describe this as evidence of flow rather than of engagement.

How engagement is understood within the conceptual framework

The European definition of *engagement* was constructed from definitions of the term found in the literature:

· ·

Engagement is a sense of involvement, choice, positive meaning and commitment while performing an occupation or activity.

· ·

This definition was constructed from five elements found in existing definitions of *engagement*:

- a sense of involvement

- a sense of choice

- a sense of positive meaning

- a sense of commitment

- while performing an occupation or activity.

A sense of involvement is the feeling of being closely concerned in or emotionally committed to a person, event or thing. For example, Doreen has a sense of involvement in the life of her village, meaning that she is committed to the welfare of the people who live there and deeply concerned about the state of the physical environment.

Having a sense of choice means being aware that what one is doing is voluntary, that it is undertaken and continued freely and autonomously. For example, Jennifer particularly enjoys writing scholarly papers when they are for her own interest and not for her employer. In both situations she could choose to stop working but, if she wants to keep her job, she sometimes has to work to someone else's agenda rather than her own, and this makes her feel less engaged in what she is doing.

A sense of positive meaning is the feeling that what one is doing is significant or important in a good way, to oneself or to others. For example, Robin is a skilled carpenter: he takes a pride in making useful and beautiful items of furniture for his friends and family. When he is painstakingly cutting a dovetail joint or carefully planing a length of wood, he knows that the recipient of the gift will appreciate the time and care he put into it, as well as valuing the object itself. This awareness is an important part of the meaning of what he is doing.

A sense of commitment is a feeling of caring, obligation or duty towards a person, activity or thing. This may be a negative sense, such as feeling that one has a duty to carry out an unpleasant task in order to meet someone else's expectations, or it may be a positive feeling, such as the joy of caring for a beloved child. The sense of commitment can vary towards different activities and towards the same activity on different occasions. For example, when Jane is preparing a dinner for her husband's business associates, she feels a strong sense of commitment to do her best. When she is cooking the evening meal for her family after a day at work she feels less committed to expending a great deal of time and effort.

The explanations given here, of the senses of involvement, choice, meaning and commitment, acknowledge that one can feel all of these in relation to people, events, activities or things. However, within the European conceptual framework, the concept of engagement refers only to the performance of an activity or occupation. Engagement is experienced during activity or occupational performance, so we can talk about someone being engaged in what she is doing, or say that a person finds engagement in physical activity to be a positive experience.

The European definition of engagement incorporates four different senses that might be experienced during activity or occupation: involvement, choice, positive meaning and commitment. It would be possible to find positive meaning in an activity but no deep sense of involvement, or to have a sense of commitment to a project but feel that one's choices about when and how to take part are limited. This means that engagement is never absolute but is always a variable state. For example, we could say that someone is deeply engaged or that a person has limited engagement in what he is doing.

RELATIONSHIPS BETWEEN TERMS REFERRING TO THE ENERGY SOURCE FOR ACTION

The three terms in the cluster of the energy source for action are closely related and, together, determine whether someone acts, what type of action is taken and the quality of the person's involvement in the activity or occupation. As described above, occupational therapists have sometimes used the terms *motivation* and *volition* synonymously. Both terms refer to reasons why people engage in activity; however, it is useful in practice to differentiate between the two concepts, as illustrated in Example 9.1.

Example 9.1: Differentiating between motivation and volition

An occupational therapist working in an acute psychiatric admission unit was aware that serious mental health problems could cause her clients to experience both low levels of motivation and problems with volition. If an individual said that he did not want to join in any activity on the ward, it was necessary for her to assess whether the issue was one of motivation or volition or both, in order to select the most appropriate intervention.

For example, Mrs Brown said that she did not want to do cookery with the therapist. On admission to the ward, she was profoundly depressed and this made her feel very tired and lacking in energy. In other words, Mrs Brown had a problem with motivation, since motivation is the energy source for action. Cookery was one of Mrs Brown's usual daily activities so the therapist reasoned that she would be willing to cook again when the depression lifted and her energy levels rose. In the meantime, the therapist tried to engage Mrs Brown in activities that demanded less energy, such as having a short conversation about the weather.

Another client, Mr Green, also said that he did not want to do cookery with the therapist. He was suffering from acute anxiety following the death of his mother, with whom he had lived all his life. The therapist reasoned that he was choosing not to cook because he had never learned to cook and had no confidence in his ability to learn how to make his own meals. She judged this to be an issue of volition, since Mr Green was choosing not to cook. However, she also felt that his ability to choose was limited by his never having cooked before and by his not knowing how to cook. In order to increase his ability to make an informed choice, that is, his volitional capacity, she persuaded him to engage in simple cooking activities, such as making toast, in order to build his confidence and skills.

Motivation is defined in the conceptual framework as a drive (that directs a person's actions towards meeting needs) and *volition* as an ability (to choose to do or continue to do something). Both of these concepts are needed to understand why a person engages in a particular action. Motivation provides the energy to act and volition directs that energy towards one activity or occupation rather than another. This is illustrated in Example 9.2.

Unlike the concepts of motivation and volition, engagement does not refer to why a person carries out an activity but to the quality of his relationship with the activity or occupation: that is, his sense of involvement, choice, positive meaning and commitment. However, a person's engagement in activity is strongly affected by his motivation and volition, as shown in Example 9.2.

Example 9.2: Interaction between motivation, volition and engagement

After a night out with friends, Liam had a good night's sleep and woke up on Sunday morning feeling full of energy. His level of motivation was high enough for him to want to engage in vigorous exercise. He considered going for a walk on the moors but decided to dig his vegetable garden instead, to prepare it for planting. In making this choice, Liam was exercising volition.

While Liam was digging, he was thinking about how beautiful the moors would look on this early spring day. He had chosen to dig the garden, and knew that he needed to get it ready for planting, but he did not feel involved in or committed to what he was doing. In other words, his engagement was not deep. He continued digging until lunchtime then, after a quick meal, went for a walk on the moors.

Shifting perspectives

Motivation, volition and engagement are abstract concepts and cannot be observed: they have to be inferred from what the individual is doing and how she is doing it. For example, if a woman freely chooses to go to a party after work, this suggests that she has both the energy (*motivation*) and the desire (*volition*) to party. The way that she behaves at the party will indicate her level of engagement in the activity: if she sits quietly with a single drink for the whole evening, declining offers to dance, we can assume that her engagement is weak. If, on the other hand, she actively solicits dancing partners, has several drinks and flirts with a number of different men, we can assume that her engagement is strong.

Although motivation and volition are different concepts there is some overlap and interplay between the two, as illustrated by Example 9.3. Both motivation and volition incorporate a sense of intention or purpose, although this is stronger in volition than in motivation. As discussed above, motivation is a drive towards meeting a particular need, therefore it directs a person towards actions that will meet that need. For example, if a man feels hungry, he experiences the urge to eat, not to go for a walk. Volition fine tunes the drive to act when there are alternative ways of meeting the need. For example, the hungry man can choose to have a sandwich, cook a meal for himself, order a takeaway or go to a restaurant.

Example 9.3: Overlap and interplay between motivation and volition

When Pauline chooses to walk to the shops, rather than catching the bus, this suggests a good level of motivation because walking demands more energy than taking the bus. However, when Pauline is tired she decides to walk to the shops anyway because she is trying to lose weight and thinks that the exercise will help. She is able to overcome her low motivation for walking because she has a strong desire to lose weight: her volition enables her to overcome her low motivation. She also finds, on many occasions, that her motivation increases once she starts walking.

Motivation is a precursor to volition: a person must have the drive to act before he can choose a course of action. Once the person has begun an activity, both motivation and volition are required in order for him to continue. For example, James is hungry (*motivation*) so he decides to order an Indian takeaway meal (*volition*). After he has eaten about half of it, he is no longer hungry but he chooses to finish one of the dishes that he particularly likes and then throw away the rest of the meal.

Engagement does not take place until the person starts to act because it is experienced while performing an occupation or activity. It is not necessary to be fully engaged in an activity in order to continue with it, if motivation and volition are strong. For example, James decides to watch a DVD while he is eating his Indian meal. He is engaged in watching the film rather than in eating.

Motivation to act is not dependent on a particular context; indeed, it is possible to experience motivation that is inappropriate to the setting, such as wanting to go to sleep during a staff meeting. It may be necessary to defer gratification of a drive until the person is in a more appropriate context. Volition is more context dependent, in that the range of choices available to a person are largely determined by the context. For example, James could not choose to have an Indian meal if this type of food was not available locally. Engagement is dependent on the activity, rather than the context, but it can be influenced by the context. If James' DVD player was broken, he might have been more engaged in eating rather than in watching a film. He writes a food column for a local paper and, when he reviews a restaurant he is much more engaged with eating.

SUMMARY

This chapter explored the terms in the energy source for action cluster that, together with the personal requisites for action cluster, make up the internal world of the performer. The terms *motivation, volition* and *engagement* are used by occupational therapists to refer to why a person performs certain activities and occupations rather than others. The chapter looked at how the three terms are used by the general public and in the occupational therapy literature. The European definitions of the terms were given, with explanations of how the definitions were constructed and what they mean. The final section considered the relationships between the three terms, highlighting the dynamic nature of those relationships.

The next chapter looks at the first cluster of terms in the external world of the performer: the social contract for action.

REFERENCES

Burke, J.P. (1977) 'A clinical perspective on motivation: pawn versus origin.' *American Journal of Occupational Therapy 31*, 4, 254–258.

Carlson, M. (1996) 'The self-perpetuation of occupations.' In R. Zemke and F. Clark (eds) *Occupational Science: The Evolving Discipline*. Philadelphia, PA: F.A. Davis.

Casson, E. (1955) 'Occupational therapy.' *Occupational Therapy 18*, 3, 98–100.

Christiansen, C. and Baum, C. (1997) 'Person-environment Occupational Performance: a conceptual model for practice.' In C. Christiansen and C. Baum (eds) *Occupational Therapy: Enabling Function and Well-being, Second Edition.* Thorofare, NJ: Slack.

Creek, J. (2003) *Occupational Therapy Defined as a Complex Intervention.* London: College of Occupational Therapists.

Creek, J. (2007) 'Engaging the reluctant client.' In J. Creek and A. Lawson-Porter (eds) *Contemporary Issues in Occupational Therapy: Reasoning and Reflection.* Chichester: Wiley.

Creek, J. (2008) 'Creative activities.' In J. Creek and L. Lougher (eds) *Occupational Therapy and Mental Health, Fourth Edition.* Edinburgh: Churchill Livingstone Elsevier.

Doble, S. (1988) 'Intrinsic motivation and clinical practice: the key to understanding the unmotivated client.' *Canadian Journal of Occupational Therapy* 55, 2, 75–80.

du Toit, V. (1991) *Patient Volition and Action in Occupational Therapy, Second Edition.* Hillbrow: Vona & Marie du Toit Foundation.

Engelhardt, H.T. (1977) 'Defining occupational therapy: the meaning of therapy and the virtues of occupation.' *American Journal of Occupational Therapy 31*, 10, 666–672.

Fleming, M.H. (1994) 'A commonsense practice in an uncommon world.' In C. Mattingly and M.H. Fleming *Clinical Reasoning: Forms of Inquiry in a Therapeutic Practice.* Philadelphia, PA: F.A. Davis.

Gelder, M., Gath, D. and Mayou, R. (1989) *Oxford Textbook of Psychiatry, Second Edition.* Oxford: Oxford University Press.

Haworth, N.A. (1933) 'Occupational therapy.' *The Lancet* Jan 21, 171–175.

Helfrich, C., Kielhofner, G. and Mattingly, C. (1994) 'Volition as narrative: understanding motivation in chronic illness.' *American Journal of Occupational Therapy* 48, 4, 311–317.

Hooper, B. and Wood, W. (2002) 'Pragmatism and structuralism in occupational therapy: the long conversation.' *American Journal of Occupational Therapy 56*, 1, 40–50.

Hughes, S. (2008) 'Approaches to severe and enduring mental illness.' In J. Creek and L. Lougher (eds) *Occupational Therapy and Mental Health, Fourth Edition.* Edinburgh: Churchill Livingstone Elsevier.

Kielhofner, G. (1980a) 'A model of human occupation, part 2: ontogenesis from the perspective of temporal adaptation.' *American Journal of Occupational Therapy 34*, 10, 657–663.

Kielhofner, G. (1980b) 'A model of human occupation, part 3: benign and vicious cycles.' *American Journal of Occupational Therapy 34*, 11, 731–737.

Kielhofner, G. and Burke, J.P. (1980) 'A model of human occupation, part 1: conceptual framework and content.' *American Journal of Occupational Therapy 34*, 9, 572–581.

Kielhofner, G., Burke, J.P. and Igi, C.H. (1980) 'A model of human occupation, part 4: assessment and intervention.' *American Journal of Occupational Therapy 34*, 12, 777–788.

Martin, M. (2009) 'Boredom as an important area of inquiry for occupational therapists.' *British Journal of Occupational Therapy 72*, 1, 40–42.

Mosey, A.C. (1986) *Psychosocial Components of Occupational Therapy.* New York: Raven Press.

Reilly, M. (1974) *Play as Exploratory Learning: Studies of Curiosity Behaviour.* Beverly Hills, CA: Sage.

Sennett, R. (2008) *The Craftsman.* London: Allen Lane.

Shorter Oxford English Dictionary, Fifth Edition (2002) Oxford: Oxford University Press.

Smith, R.E. (1993) *Psychology.* Minneapolis/St. Paul: West Publishing Company.

Stewart, P. and Craik, C. (2007) 'Occupation, mental illness and medium security: exploring time-use in forensic regional secure units.' *British Journal of Occupational Therapy 70*, 10, 416–425.

Timmons, A. and MacDonald, E. (2008) '"Alchemy and magic": the experience of using clay for people with chronic illness and disability.' *British Journal of Occupational Therapy 71*, 3, 86–94.

World Health Organization (2001) *ICF: International Classification of Functioning, Disability and Health.* Geneva: World Health Organization.

CHAPTER 10

SOCIAL CONTRACT FOR ACTION

INTRODUCTION

The last two chapters discussed the meanings of two clusters of terms that occupational therapists use to refer to the internal world of the performer: the personal requisites for action and the energy source for action. This chapter and the next one will explore the meanings of the terms in the two clusters that make up the external world of the performer: the social contract for action and the place for action.

The social contract for action refers to the influences that other people have on what activities and occupations a person performs, how frequently they are performed and the quality of the performer's engagement. The cluster is made up of three terms: *role, participation* and *task*. A definition of *task* was given in Chapter 4, where it was explained that occupational therapists use the term with two different meanings. The second definition is given in this chapter.

ROLE

This section explores what the word *role* means in common usage and the different ways in which it is used. It then looks at how occupational therapists have used the term and at how it is defined in the conceptual framework.

What role means in common usage

The word *role* is commonly used in English in a variety of contexts, especially in the context of play or film acting. One of the definitions of the word given in the *Shorter Oxford English Dictionary* (2002) is: 'an actor's part in a play, film, etc.'. So, we might say that Vivienne Leigh was superb in the role of Scarlett O'Hara in the film of *Gone with the Wind*, or that Val Kilmer took over the role of Batman from Michael Keaton in the third film about the superhero.

The *Shorter Oxford English Dictionary* (2002) gives two further definitions of *role*:

1. The part played or assumed by a person in society, life etc.

2. The characteristic or expected function of a person or thing, especially in a particular setting or environment.

The first of these definitions is close in meaning to the way that the term is used in the disciplines of sociology and anthropology: '*Roles* are those parts of individual and group behaviour which are given definition and context by the particular society of which one is a member' (Mangen 1982, p.8). This definition incorporates the idea that a role has both personal and social aspects. An individual takes on and enacts a role, but society is the context in which roles are assigned and played, and social expectations determine to a large extent how each role is played.

The word is also used in this first meaning in the context of psychodrama or dramatherapy, where we might talk about role-playing, about someone acting out a role, or about two people reversing their usual roles. In group psychotherapy, the ways that members behave in the group can be understood in terms of the roles that they take on, such as harmonizer, follower or energizer (Cole 2008, p.324).

In the second meaning of the word, we might talk about a man taking the dominant role in his marriage, or about a shop steward taking a key role in pay negotiations in the workplace.

Both of these *Shorter Oxford English Dictionary* definitions are relevant to the way in which the term *role* is used in the conceptual framework.

How occupational therapists use the term role

The concept of *role* is an important one in occupational therapy theory:

> Roles...outline the nature of occupational performance at various points in time. Thus, it can be asserted that occupational performance

deficits have meaning principally in the context of an individual's role responsibilities. (Christiansen and Baum 1997, p.56)

Many attempts have been made to differentiate *role* from *occupation*. As discussed in Chapter 4, Hagedorn (2000) described a taxonomy of occupation in which the highest level consists of social roles, 'which direct the individual's engagement in certain activities or tasks related to the role over extended periods of time' (p.26), and occupations, which are 'a form of human endeavour which provides longitudinal organization of time and effort in a person's life' (p.309). However, these definitions do not make a clear difference between a role and an occupation.

An early occupational therapy model, the model of human occupation, located roles within the habituation sub-system, along with habits (Kielhofner 1992). In this model, roles are defined as 'images that persons hold about the positions they occupy in various social groups and of the obligations that go along with those positions' (p.158). A later version of the model described a role as:

> a kind of framework for looking out on the world and for engaging in occupation. Thus, when one is engaging in an occupation within a given role, it may be reflected in how the person dresses, the demeanour of the person, the content of one's actions and so on. We need only reflect on how we behave within our worker role versus our role as a parent, spouse or friend to see how the role we are in shapes our behaviour. (Forsyth and Kielhofner 2006, p.74)

Creek (2008, p.40) attempted to clarify the difference between role and occupation by suggesting that:

> An occupation and a social role may share the same name, although a role is more likely to be described by a noun and an occupation by a verb. For example, *mother* is a role while *mothering* is an occupation. The concept of occupation is mainly concerned with the actions that a person takes to achieve his purposes while the concept of role is mainly concerned with social expectations and the mechanisms by which society shapes the actions of individuals.

Occupational therapists talk about role areas in a similar way to occupational performance areas, including family roles, social roles and even occupational roles: for example, 'specific occupational roles are not limited to paid employment and, therefore, can include housewife, student, preschooler, or retiree' (Reed and Sanderson 1992, p.56).

Occupational therapists also write about their professional role, either expressing concern that it is poorly understood (Creek 1998; Williams and Bannigan 2008), attempting to delineate the professional role of the occupational therapist (Fleming and Mattingly 1994; Pollard, Sakellariou and Kronenberg 2009) or describing the role of the occupational therapist in different fields of practice (Culverhouse and Bibby 2008; Joss 2007; Pope, Davys and Taylor 2008). Ormston (2008, p.232) pointed out that 'the role balance health professionals are expected to achieve is highly complex' and that the many roles of the occupational therapist in the field of mental health include: manager, researcher, clinician, colleague and generic mental health worker.

How role is understood within the conceptual framework

The European definition of *role* was constructed from existing definitions of the term:

· ·

A *role* is the social and cultural norms and expectations of occupational performance that are associated with the individual's social and personal identity.

· ·

This definition is constructed from seven elements that were found within definitions of *role* in the literature:

- social norms

- social expectations

- cultural norms

- cultural expectations

- of occupational performance

- associated with an individual's social identity

- associated with an individual's personal identity.

Social means 'connected with the functions and structures necessary to membership of a group or society', and norms are 'what is expected or regarded as normal' (*Shorter Oxford English Dictionary* 2002). In the context of the European definition, therefore, social norms are those actions regarded as normal within a particular group or society. For example, in the UK it is a social norm that the audience at an opera do not applaud during an act but wait until the end.

Expectations are preconceived ideas about what is going to happen, therefore social expectations are the ideas that members of a particular group or society have about how an individual is going to act. For example, in the UK there is an expectation that people will queue to be served at a post office counter, rather than pushing to the front.

Cultural means pertaining to the distinctive outlook of a society or civilization, therefore cultural norms are the actions regarded as normal from the perspective of a particular society or civilization. For example, in some cultures it is the norm for elderly people to be cared for at home by their relatives, while in others it is the norm for people to go into residential care when they are no longer able to look after themselves.

Cultural expectations are the distinctive ideas about how an individual will act that are characteristic of a particular society or civilization. For example, in some cultures there is an expectation that a woman will be a virgin until she marries.

Occupational performance was defined in Chapter 5 as choosing, organizing and carrying out occupations in interaction with the environment. For example, Kate decides to take her husband to the theatre as a birthday surprise. She chooses a play that she thinks he will enjoy, books the tickets, lets him know that they will be going out that evening and accompanies him to the theatre. Choosing, organizing and carrying out these actions add up to a piece of occupational performance.

Identity is those characteristics which determine that a person is that specified unique person (*Shorter Oxford English Dictionary* 2002). Social identity is the characteristics that are ascribed to a person, or viewed as representative of him, within a particular group or society. For example, within his church community, John is seen as honest, loyal, reliable and hard-working: these characteristics largely constitute his social identity. Personal identity is the characteristics that a person experiences as constant in his personality, which give him a sense of sameness and continuity. For example, John is not comfortable with too many changes, which make him feel anxious, he prefers the company of people he knows, he likes to feel in control of any job that he undertakes and he is deeply attached to his family: these characteristics form part of his personal identity.

Within the European conceptual framework, therefore, a *role* is the occupational performance that is expected or required of a particular person within a particular social context. For example, the way that Clare performs her role of mother is shaped by her own and her social group's ideas of what a mother should do.

This section has offered a brief discussion of an important term about which much has been written. The interested reader is recommended to explore the writings of other disciplines, such as sociology and anthropology, on the concept of *role*.

PARTICIPATION

This section begins with an exploration of what the word *participation* means in common usage and the ways in which it is used. It then looks at how occupational therapists have used the term and at how it is defined within the conceptual framework.

What participation means in common usage

The *Shorter Oxford English Dictionary* (2002) gives four definitions of *participation*:

1. The action or fact of having or forming part of.

2. The fact or condition of sharing in common.

3. The action or an act of taking part with others (in an action or matter).

4. The active involvement of members of a community or organization in decisions which affect them.

The writer and philosopher, Francis Bacon, was using the word in its first sense when he wrote 'Poesy was ever thought to have some participation of divineness' (*Oxford Dictionary of Quotations* 1990), meaning that poetry is partly divine. The word is not often used in this way in modern English.

The word is being given its second meaning when we talk about the participation of millions in grieving for Diana, Princess of Wales, after her death in 1997.

We are using the word in its third sense when we talk about the participation of union members in a strike, and in its fourth sense when we say that there was full participation in the ballot on strike action.

The term *participation* has come to be used more widely in health and social care settings following the publication, in 2001, of the *International*

Classification of Functioning, Disability and Health (ICF) (World Health Organization 2001). In this classification, participation is defined as 'involvement in a life situation' (p.10) and covers aspects of individual functioning from a societal perspective. When an individual experiences problems with involvement in life situations, this is known as participation restriction.

How occupational therapists use the term participation

The way that occupational therapists use the term *participation* has changed over the years, influenced by the way that it is defined in the ICF (World Health Organization 2001). They have written both about the client's participation in therapeutic activities and, more recently, about encouraging participation in the life of the community. For example, Hagedorn (2000, p.116) described one of the skills of the occupational therapist as 'the ability to motivate participation' in therapeutic activity. Six years later, Forsyth and Kielhofner (2006, p.77) wrote that 'participation refers to engagement in work, play or activities of daily living that are part of one's sociocultural context and that are desired and/or necessary to one's well-being'.

Polgar and Landry (2004) wrote about both participation in occupation and occupation as a means for participation in life. They asserted that 'participation in occupation defines who we are, either as individuals or as members of our communities' (p.197).

In 1994, Fleming wrote about occupational therapists placing special importance on the client's '*willing participation* in action taking and meaning-making' (p.101), implying that the therapist wants to encourage the person's sense of connectedness to the world. In a similar vein, Creek (2007, p.127) wrote that 'active participation by the individual in the process of therapy, as opposed to passive compliance, increases his choice, autonomy, responsibility for outcomes and control over his care'.

Creek (2008) differentiated between the concepts of *engagement* and *participation*, arguing that it is possible for a person to participate in an activity without being fully engaged, that is, without feeling fully involved and committed. However, engagement in activity is not possible without participation. This suggests that there are degrees of participation, from the peripheral participation of a spectator watching a replay of a football match on television to the full participation of a player on the field.

During recent years, occupational therapists have begun to write about the conditions that can inhibit full participation in occupations or life situations, for example, 'poverty restricted opportunities for participation in certain occupations' (Fourie *et al.* 2004, p.73).

How participation is understood within the conceptual framework

The European definition of *participation* is partly constructed from the ICF definition but adds two elements taken from definitions in the occupational therapy literature:

···

Participation is involvement in life situations through activity within a social context.

···

The definition is made up of four elements:

• involvement

• in life situations

• through activity

• within a social context.

The first two elements of the definition were taken from the ICF definition of participation: 'involvement in a life situation' (World Health Organization 2001, p.10). Involvement is defined in Chapter 9 as the feeling of being closely concerned in or emotionally committed to a person, event or thing. Life situations are the context for performance, including social and physical environments and events.

The European definition of participation has added two further elements to the ICF definition. People are involved in life situations through activity, because activity is the interface between the individual and the environment, the means by which he influences and is influenced by the external world.

Every human being develops throughout his life via his *activity*, involving the perception of capacities and relationships in his environment and the acquisition of new skills through action. Through his actions, the person also changes his environment, at the same time developing and changing his own action possibilities. (Fortmeier and Thanning 2002, pp.27–28)

The second element added to the ICF definition is 'within a social context'. The concept of *context* is discussed in Chapter 11, where it is defined as the relationships between the environment, personal factors and events that influence the meaning of a task, activity or occupation for the performer. A *social context* is, therefore, the functions and structures that accompany membership of a group or society and that influence what an activity or occupation means to the performer. When a person participates in an occupation, it is always within a social context, even when no one else is present, because the occupations that are chosen and the way that they are performed are strongly influenced by social and cultural norms and expectations.

TASK

As explained in Chapter 4, occupational therapists use the word *task* in two ways. In Chapter 4, a task was defined as a series of structured steps (actions and/or thoughts) intended to accomplish the performance of an activity. In this chapter, an alternative meaning of the word is explored.

What task means in common usage

The *Shorter Oxford English Dictionary* (2002) offers several definitions of the word *task*, including 'a lesson to be learned or prepared' and 'a tribute'. Four definitions are relevant to the way the word is defined in the conceptual framework:

1. A piece of work imposed on or undertaken by a person.

2. A fixed quantity of labour to be performed by a person.

3. The work allotted as a duty to a specific person.

4. A thing that has to be done, *esp.* one involving labour or difficulty.

We are using the word in its first sense when we say that a librarian was given the task of cataloguing a delivery of new books. The word is being used in its second sense when we say that the librarian knew he could not go home until the task of cataloguing the latest delivery of books was completed. In the third sense of the word, we might say that the task of cataloguing new books was a major part of the librarian's job and, in the fourth sense, that the librarian found cataloguing books to be an onerous task. The words task and job are sometimes used interchangeably, for example, we could say that the librarian was given the task of cataloguing books or the job of cataloguing books.

In common usage, the word task often has a negative connotation, as in 'an unpleasant task' or an 'unwelcome task', although it would not be incorrect to talk about 'an enjoyable task'.

A further definition of task comes from its use in the discipline of psychology: 'a piece of work or an exercise given to a subject in a psychological test or experiment' (*Shorter Oxford English Dictionary* 2002). For example, in a verbal conditioning experiment, 'the subjects' task was to make up a series of sentences' (Smith 1993, p.286).

How occupational therapists use the term *task*

As discussed in Chapter 4, occupational therapists commonly use the word *task* to describe a component or stage of an activity, defining it as 'a constituent part of an activity' (Creek 2002, p.588). However, they also use it with the meaning explored in this chapter: a thing that has to be done or work allotted to a person. For example, 'Everyday routines or tasks maintain the person in a positive relation with both the objective, and subjective social world' (Fleming 1994, p.106).

The word *task* is frequently used in connection with group work, for example, 'When members deviate from the group tasks or goal, the occupational therapy leader needs to redirect' (Cole 2008, p.322).

Some writers have referred to the tasks of the occupational therapist, meaning the actions that she is expected to carry out as part of her job. For example, 'in considering the work performed by a staff member, first it is necessary to identify the specific tasks that he or she performs and to check whether this information has been made available to the worker' (Willson 1996, p.256).

Occupational therapists also talk about multitasking, meaning carrying out several tasks together, dovetailing and prioritizing them to make the most effective use of time (Cook 2008). This concept has been explored in the discipline of occupational science, where multitasking has been described as 'doing a variety of tasks in an enfolded manner' (Bateson 1996, p.8).

How task is understood within the conceptual framework

The European definition of *task* is constructed from definitions found in the literature:

> ···
>
> A *task* is a piece of work the individual is expected to do.
>
> ···

This definition is made up of two elements:

- a piece of work

- the individual is expected to do.

Work is 'purposive action involving effort or exertion' (*Shorter Oxford English Dictionary* 2002). To be expected to do something means that others are looking to the individual to act, as a duty or requirement. So, in this sense, a task is an action involving effort that the individual is required to do in order to meet the expectations of others. For example, each member of the ENOTHE terminology group took on the task of finding a publisher for the conceptual framework in her or his own country.

RELATIONSHIPS BETWEEN TERMS

The three terms discussed in this chapter represent aspects of the social context in which people perform their occupations, activities and tasks, and which shapes how those occupations, activities and tasks are performed. *Role* refers to the social and cultural norms and expectations that are part of each person's life context. *Participation* refers more broadly to involvement with the social context of performance, which consists of all the functions and structures that are part of membership of a society. *Task* refers to effort the individual is required to make in order to meet the expectations of others.

All three terms incorporate both society's norms and/or expectations of individual performance and the individual's experience of those expectations. The concepts of *role* and *participation* imply individual choice: to some extent we can choose which roles we take on and the degree to which we participate in society. The concept of *task* carries more of an implication of coercion, although tasks may be undertaken willingly. Being forced to carry out tasks that the individual does not want to perform can lead to occupational alienation. For example, a prisoner or a detained patient is not only separated from his normal daily activities and routines but may be expected to carry out new activities and routines that he finds distasteful or degrading, such as slopping out his cell or queuing for medication.

The concepts of *role* and *task* both refer to the expectations of others and the individual's internalization of those expectations. However, *role* encompasses social and cultural expectations about all aspects of occupational performance while *task* refers specifically to expectations about a discrete piece of work. The concept of *participation* focuses on the individual's experience, with the implication that this experience is shaped by the social context of performance. The term is used to refer both to the individual's experience of performing an occupation or activity and to his experience of taking part in the life of the community.

Example 10.1 illustrates how the three concepts contribute to our understanding of the ways that performance, and the performer's experience, are shaped by the social context.

Example 10.1: How the experience of performance is shaped by social context

Mrs Bright was admitted to hospital for assessment following a fall that resulted in mild hypothermia. She had been unable to get up by herself and was on the floor for several hours before a neighbour found her. While in hospital, she refused to join in any of the activities suggested by the occupational therapist, saying that she was in hospital for a rest. She believed that the role of the patient is to rest in order to get well as quickly as possible.

The multidisciplinary team thought that the fall might have been due to Mrs Bright not eating properly and they were concerned that she would relapse if she went home. They asked the occupational therapist to do a meal planning and cooking assessment to find out whether Mrs Bright was able to manage on her own. Mrs Bright did not want to have her cooking skills assessed but she thought that she would not be allowed to go home unless she completed the task successfully, so she agreed to plan and cook lunch for herself and the therapist.

The session was a success and the occupational therapist suggested that Mrs Bright should be allowed to go home, with one or more follow-up visits to see how she was managing. The therapist then made sure that she dropped in at lunchtime one day, to find out if Mrs Bright was cooking and eating a balanced meal.

To her surprise, the therapist found Mrs Bright eating a freshly cooked meal with two friends. They told her that, since their husbands died, they had got into the habit of cooking for each other once a week. They rotated the days so that each person cooked Sunday dinner once every three weeks. Cooking and eating with friends was an important aspect of Mrs Bright's participation in the life of her community.

In Mrs Bright's social and cultural world, cooking is not part of the role of patient: cooking for the purpose of having one's competence assessed is a task, but cooking for friends is a form of participation.

Shifting perspectives

All the terms in the social contract for action cluster represent concepts that give meaning and purpose to human performance. A role gives meaning to occupational performance through the social and cultural norms and expectations that it embodies, and it confers social identity and status. For example, when an occupational therapist is performing her job, some of its meaning comes from her awareness of the social status of her role. Some roles have higher status than others in a particular society: the role of occupational therapist has a lower social status than that of doctor in the UK but a higher social status than the role of ward clerk.

The concept of participation implies that a life situation has meaning for a person: if a situation does not have meaning for the individual, he will not feel involved and his participation will be more peripheral. Since roles give meaning to occupational performance, they influence the extent of an individual's participation in life situations.

The meaning and purpose of a task come from the expectations of others. The task may be a one-off, such as clearing a blocked gutter, or it may be part of a role, for example, a ward clerk has the task of filing patients' notes.

Roles and tasks are abstract and non-observable: they can only be inferred from watching a person's performance or asking what meaning and purpose it has for him. For example, if we see someone clearing the gutter, we cannot immediately know if he is experiencing the action as a task, which is a piece of work he is expected to do, or as a freely chosen activity. Participation is more easily inferred from observing the context in which a person performs an activity or occupation although, as described above, there are different forms of participation, as illustrated in Example 10.2.

Example 10.2: Forms of participation

Many people participate in a professional game of football, although they may do so in different ways and with varying degrees of involvement. The players on the field are participating actively, the substitutes waiting on the side less so. The sports commentators who cover the match are participating as actively as the players but in a different way. The spectators at the match are participating more immediately than the people in a pub who are watching it on television in real time. They, in turn, are experiencing a greater degree of involvement than the man who watches the highlights of the match on television that evening.

The participation of the groundsmen who are responsible for keeping the pitch in good condition is mostly over before the match starts, although they may have to be on hand in case they are needed. A groundsman may also choose to participate in the match in a different way by becoming a spectator. The speculators who finance the two teams participate in the sport in a different way from the players, but they may also be spectators.

Role, participation and task are all dependent on the social context in which performance takes place, and are shaped by that context. Participation and task are also dependent on a physical environment, in that they involve performance. In contrast, a role can exist independently of its enactment: the householder still has that role even when he is at work.

SUMMARY

This chapter explored the terms used by occupational therapists to refer to the social context that shapes how people perform their tasks, activities and occupations. These terms are *task*, *role* and *participation*. The chapter considered how these terms are used by the general public and in the occupational therapy literature. The European definitions of the terms were given, with explanations of how the definitions were constructed and what they mean. The final section considered the relationships between the three terms, highlighting the dynamic nature of those relationships.

The next chapter looks at the second and final cluster of terms in the external world of the performer: the *place for action*. This cluster is the last of the eight clusters that make up the European conceptual framework for occupational therapy.

REFERENCES

Bateson, M.C. (1996) 'Enfolded activity and the concept of occupation.' In R. Zemke and F. Clark (eds) *Occupational Science: The Evolving Discipline.* Philadelphia, PA: F.A. Davis.

Christiansen, C. and Baum, C. (1997) 'Person-environment occupational performance.' In C. Christiansen and C. Baum (eds) *Occupational Therapy: Enabling Function and Well-being, Second Edition.* Thorofare, NJ: Slack.

Cole, M.B. (2008) 'Client-centred groups.' In J. Creek and L. Lougher (eds) *Occupational Therapy and Mental Health, Fourth Edition*. Edinburgh: Churchill Livingstone Elsevier.

Cook, C. (2008) 'An exploration of the neural control of multitasking and the implications for practice.' *British Journal of Occupational Therapy 71*, 6, 241–247.

Creek, J. (1998) 'Communicating the nature and purpose of occupational therapy.' In J. Creek (ed.) *Occupational Therapy: New Perspectives*. London: Whurr.

Creek, J. (ed.) (2002) *Occupational Therapy and Mental Health, Third Edition*. Edinburgh: Churchill Livingstone.

Creek, J. (2007) 'Engaging the reluctant client.' In J. Creek and A. Lawson-Porter (eds) *Contemporary Issues in Occupational Therapy: Reasoning and Reflection*. Chichester: Wiley.

Creek, J. (2008) 'The knowledge base of occupational therapy.' In J. Creek and L. Lougher (eds) *Occupational Therapy and Mental Health, Fourth Edition*. Edinburgh: Churchill Livingstone Elsevier.

Culverhouse, J. and Bibby, P.F. (2008) 'Occupational therapy and care coordination: the challenges faced by occupational therapists in community mental health settings.' *British Journal of Occupational Therapy 71*, 11, 496–498.

Fleming, M.H. (1994) 'A commonsense practice in an uncommon world.' In C. Mattingly, and M.H. Fleming *Clinical Reasoning: Forms of Inquiry in a Therapeutic Practice*. Philadelphia, PA: F.A. Davis.

Fleming, M.H. and Mattingly, C. (1994) 'The underground practice.' In C. Mattingly and M.H. Fleming *Clinical Reasoning: Forms of Inquiry in a Therapeutic Practice*. Philadelphia, PA: F.A. Davis.

Forsyth, K. and Kielhofner, G. (2006) 'The model of human occupation: integrating theory into practice and practice into theory.' In E.A.S. Duncan (ed.) *Foundations for Practice in Occupational Therapy, Fourth Edition*. Edinburgh: Elsevier Churchill Livingstone.

Fortmeier, S. and Thanning, G. (2002) *From the Patient's Point of View: An Activity Theory Approach to Occupational Theory*. Copenhagen: Ergoterapeutforeningen.

Fourie, M., Galvaan, R. and Beeton, H. (2004) 'The impact of poverty: potential lost.' In R. Watson and L. Swartz (eds) *Transformation through Occupation*. London: Whurro.

Hagedorn, R. (2000) *Tools for Practice in Occupational Therapy: A Structured Approach to Core Skills and Processes*. Edinburgh: Churchill Livingstone.

Joss, M. (2007) 'The importance of job analysis in occupational therapy.' *British Journal of Occupational Therapy 70*, 7, 301–303.

Kielhofner, G. (1992) *Conceptual Foundations of Occupational Therapy*. Philadelphia, PA: F.A. Davis.

Mangen, S.P. (1982) *Sociology and Mental Health: An Introduction for Nurses and Other Care-givers*. Edinburgh: Churchill Livingstone.

Ormston, C. (2008) 'Roles and settings.' In J. Creek and L. Lougher (eds) *Occupational Therapy and Mental Health, Fourth Edition*. Edinburgh: Churchill Livingstone Elsevier.

Oxford Dictionary of Quotations (1990) Oxford: Oxford University Press.

Polgar, J.M. and Landry, J.E. (2004) 'Occupations as a means for individual and group participation in life.' In C.H. Christiansen and E.A. Townsend (eds) *Introduction to Occupation: The Art and Science of Living*. Upper Saddle River, NJ: Prentice Hall.

Pollard, N., Sakellariou, D. and Kronenberg, F. (2009) 'Political competence in occupational therapy.' In N. Pollard, D. Sakellariou and F. Kronenberg (eds) *A Political Practice of Occupational Therapy*. Edinburgh: Churchill Livingstone Elsevier.

Pope, K., Davys, D. and Taylor, J. (2008) 'Professionalism, personal taste and social inclusion: does it matter what clients wear?' *British Journal of Occupational Therapy 71*, 4, 165–167.

Reed, K.L. and Sanderson, S.N. (1992) *Concepts of Occupational Therapy, Third Edition*. Baltimore, MD: Williams & Wilkins.

Shorter Oxford English Dictionary, Fifth Edition (2002) Oxford: Oxford University Press.

Smith, R.E. (1993) *Psychology.* Minneapolis/St. Paul: West Publishing.

Williams, H. and Bannigan, K. (2008) 'A simple trick to market ourselves.' *British Journal of Occupational Therapy 71,* 6, 225.

Willson, M. (1996) *Occupational Therapy in Short-term Psychiatry, Third Edition.* Edinburgh: Churchill Livingstone.

World Health Organization (2001) *ICF: International Classification of Functioning, Disability and Health.* Geneva: World Health Organization.

CHAPTER 11

PLACE FOR ACTION

INTRODUCTION

This chapter discusses the second cluster of terms that, together with the social contract for action, make up the external world of the performer. The place for action consists of three terms: *setting, environment* and *context*. These are all terms used to refer to the place where tasks, activities and occupations are performed. They are often used interchangeably but this chapter suggests that the terms can be differentiated and that there is practical use in making the distinction.

SETTING

The term *setting* is used by occupational therapists less frequently and with a narrower meaning than the other two terms in the cluster. This section begins with an introduction to what the word means in common usage, then discusses the ways in which occupational therapists have used it, finishing with an explanation of the European definition of *setting*.

What setting means in common usage

The noun *setting* has several meanings in common usage. It can mean 'the manner or position in which something is set', 'a person's or thing's immediate environment or surroundings' or 'a place or time in or at which a story, play, scene, etc. is represented as happening' (*Shorter Oxford English Dictionary* 2002).

In the first meaning of the word, we might say that a sunny window sill is the perfect setting for an exotic plant. The second dictionary definition comes close to the meaning of the term within the European conceptual framework. We might say, for example, that the kitchen was an incongruous setting for John's proposal of marriage to his girlfriend. We are using the word in its third meaning when we say that the Regency period provides the setting for many of Georgette Heyer's novels.

The implication in all these examples is that a setting is not neutral but may be appropriate or inappropriate for the objects, people and events that it contains.

How occupational therapists use the term setting

The word *setting* is not generally seen as a specialist occupational therapy term and does not appear in the index or glossary of any major occupational therapy textbook. However, it is widely used to refer to the places where occupational therapy interventions take place, such as hospital settings or community settings. For example, Ormston (2008, p.215) wrote that 'Occupational therapists based in inpatient settings and longer term treatment/care settings have to continue to adapt to the changing needs of this population'.

Howe and Briggs (1982) described an ecological systems model for occupational therapy in which the individual lives in 'a series of nested environmental layers, each embedded within the next' (p.323). These layers are the individual's inner life space, the immediate setting, social networks and institutions and an outer ideological layer, which 'consists of societal and social values' (p.324). The immediate setting includes 'a person's residence, neighbourhood, family, and the other people with whom he or she is in continuing contact' (p.323).

How setting is understood within the conceptual framework

The European definition of *setting* was constructed from definitions of the term found in the literature:

• •

The *setting* is the immediate surroundings that influence task, activity or occupational performance.

• •

This definition includes two elements taken from existing definitions of *setting*:

- the immediate surroundings

- that influence task, activity or occupational performance.

Immediate means 'not separated by any intervening agent or medium' or 'nearest, next, or close in space or order' (*Shorter Oxford English Dictionary* 2002). For example, a person might talk about the buildings and streets around his house as the 'immediate neighbourhood'. Surroundings are 'those things which surround or are in the vicinity of a person or thing' (*ibid.*). For example, we might say that a picnic site in a wooded valley is located in beautiful surroundings, or that a writer does not notice his surroundings when he is absorbed in a piece of work. The immediate surroundings are those things that directly encircle or enclose a person or thing, such as the walls, doors, windows, fittings, decorations, furnishings and other objects that make up the room in which she is sitting.

Influence is 'an action exerted...by indirect means by one person or thing on another so as to cause changes in conduct, development, conditions, etc.' (*Shorter Oxford English Dictionary* 2002). When we talk about the influence of Picasso on later generations of artists, we mean that his work informs what they do in some way. As discussed in Chapter 5, the terms task, activity and occupational performance mean choosing, organizing and carrying out a task, activity or occupation in interaction with the environment. So, an influence on performance is something which changes that performance by indirect means. For example, images of very thin models in fashion magazines may influence girls to eat less in order to lose weight.

We can apply the term *setting*, in the sense of the European definition, to any of the immediate surroundings that influence any form of task, activity or occupational performance, such as the treatment setting, the work setting or the community setting.

ENVIRONMENT

The concept of *environment* became increasingly important to occupational therapists in the latter half of the twentieth century, as the focus of their work shifted from working with patients in hospital to ensuring that people are able to remain safely in their own homes, workplaces and communities. Indeed, most would argue that 'the individual cannot be understood outside the context of his environment' (Mosey 1986, p.171).

This section discusses the meaning of the word *environment* in common usage, explores the ways in which occupational therapists use the term and explains the European definition.

What environment means in common usage

According to the *Shorter Oxford English Dictionary* (2002), *environment* is 'the set of circumstances or conditions, esp. physical conditions, in which a person or community lives, works, develops, etc'. The *Dictionary* also offers *setting* and *context* as synonyms for environment.

The word *environment* is used especially to refer to physical conditions. For example, when we talk about the natural environment or the built environment, we are usually referring to the physical surroundings. In recent years, there has been great concern about the state of the environment, meaning the physical world, due to the negative effects of pollution, over-cultivation and global warming.

The environment can be the immediate surroundings, such as the school environment, or a much wider area, such as the global environment. When the word is used to refer to circumstances or conditions other than physical ones, it is often prefixed with an adjective: for example, the working environment, which might include other people and their expectations in addition to the physical place of work.

Two publications from the World Health Organization emphasize the importance of the environment to health and function. The *Ottawa Charter for Health Promotion* (World Health Organization 1986) states that an ability to cope with the environment is a prerequisite for good health and well-being. The *International Classification of Functioning, Disability and Health* (ICF) (World Health Organization 2001) describes environmental factors as some of the contextual factors that influence functioning and disability, along with personal factors. Environmental factors 'make up the physical, social and attitudinal environment in which people live and conduct their lives' (p.10).

How occupational therapists use the term environment

In 1972, an American occupational therapist, Helen Dunning, suggested that occupational therapists have a role as 'environmental managers' (p.292), referring to the treatment environment, not to the patient's own living or working environment. Dunning argued that occupational therapists, in order to understand human behaviour and to be able to change it through occupation, need a deep knowledge of the relationship between person and environment. The treatment environment consists of 'space, people, and task': 'Space is designed to promote stimulation. People are arranged to encourage social interaction. Tasks are used to develop skills' (Dunning 1972, p.292).

During the 1980s, occupational therapists began 'to move away from the dominant biomedical conceptual models, which are centered on the individual, to the contemporary perspective of social change which centers on the environment' (Fougeyrollas 1997, p.382). For example, Llorens (1984) suggested that the individual himself should be seen as a 'first level environment':

> As occupational therapists, we have identified interior environmental factors related to biological, psychophysiological, and sociological functioning that can be changed by administration or prescription of activity... The integrity of the individual and the intrapersonal environment are critical to the individual's ability to function adaptively in the second and third level environments of family/spouse/partner interactions and community relationships. (*ibid.*,p.29)

As occupational therapists are increasingly using a language of occupation to describe their theory and practice, further models have been developed to explain the relationship between the person, the environment and occupation. For example, the Canadian Model of Occupational Performance (Canadian Association of Occupational Therapists 1993) describes an interaction between occupational performance, the environment and the individual's performance components, while two American occupational therapists proposed a person–environment occupational performance model (Christiansen and Baum 1997). Within these models, the environment is described as having as much impact on the individual's occupations as his performance capacities:

> The *environment* shapes and is shaped by a person's participation in occupations. If the environment affords opportunities for participation in many occupations, the individual or community then has the choice to determine the nature of that participation. (Polgar and Landry 2004, p.203)

The interaction between person and environment works both ways, with the individual's occupations both changing the environment and enabling her adaptation or adjustment to it: 'through occupations, a person may adapt to the environment or adapt the environment to the person' (Reed and Sanderson 1992, p.87).

Different types of environment, or ways of classifying the environment, have been proposed, such as:

- cultural, social and physical environments (Mosey 1986)

- social, political, economic, institutional and cultural environments (Law *et al.* 1997)

- physical, social, cultural, economic and political environments (Creek 2008).

The occupational scientist, Ann Wilcock (1998), developed an occupational theory of health in which she argued that people's occupational behaviour is the result of natural selection, as humans have learned from and adapted to their environments through occupation. Environments differ according to ecological, cultural, social and familial factors, and children learn how to survive in the particular environments in which they grow up.

Hagedorn (2001) described environmental analysis and adaptation as core processes in occupational therapy. Three processes are involved:

- Content analysis – Analysis of the content of the environment means looking at what is there 'at work, at home, at school, in an institution, out of doors, in a public place [to] provide information on the causes of problems for the individual, explanations for behaviour or ideas or suggestions for therapeutic modifications' (p.44).

- Demand analysis – Environmental demand, or press, is the elements of the environment that produce expectations for specific, appropriate occupational performance. Analysis of environmental demand 'explores the psychological, cultural and social impact of the environment with reference to the effects of these factors in facilitating or inhibiting participation in occupations and activities' (p.44).

- Adaptation – The therapist may 'alter, remove or add to elements of the environment…in order to remove obstacles to performance or enhance the opportunities for performance, learning or development' (p.45).

Some occupational therapists have combined the words *environment* and *context* into *environmental context,* in an attempt to create 'a vocabulary for describing the immediate, more proximal environments in which we interact with objects in the physical-spatial world' (Henderson 2001, p.421). This will be further explored in the section on *context.*

How environment is understood within the conceptual framework

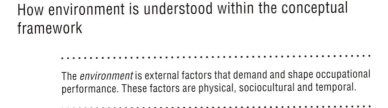

The *environment* is external factors that demand and shape occupational performance. These factors are physical, sociocultural and temporal.

This definition was constructed from six elements found in existing definitions of *environment* in the occupational therapy literature:

- external factors

- demand occupational performance

- shape occupational performance

- physical factors

- sociocultural factors

- temporal factors.

A *factor* is 'a circumstance, fact or influence which tends to produce a result' (*Shorter Oxford English Dictionary* 2002). External factors are those circumstances situated outside the person that tend to determine whether and how he performs. For example, Mike goes for a walk twice a day because he has a dog. The dog is an external factor influencing Mike's walking performance. Some definitions of environment found in the occupational therapy literature incorporate internal factors, but these are in a minority and internal factors have not been included in this definition.

A demand is an insistent or authoritative request or requirement. To demand occupational performance is to require that a person chooses, organizes and carries out an occupation. Mike's dog demands to be taken for a walk by whining and scratching at the door. Inanimate features of the environment can also demand performance, for example, walking on rough ground places demands on the body for balance and coordination.

To shape something is to form or change it into a particular configuration. To shape occupational performance means to determine how a person chooses, organizes and carries out an occupation. The weather shapes Mike's occupational performance by influencing where he takes the dog for its morning and evening walks, how quickly they walk and how long they stay out.

Physical factors are material objects, situated outside the person, that tend to determine whether and how he performs. When Mike lived in a city, he drove to a park to walk his dog: the narrow pavements and heavy traffic were physical factors that influenced him not to walk in the streets around his house.

Sociocultural factors are the circumstances and influences arising from the group or community in which the person is situated that tend to determine whether and how he performs. Now that Mike has moved to the country he can walk in the fields, but he keeps his dog on the lead when there are livestock in a field and he always closes gates behind him. The expectations of local farmers, that walkers will conform to the countryside code, are a sociocultural factor that influences how Mike performs his daily walks.

Temporal factors are circumstances relating to time which tend to determine whether and how a person performs, such as time of day and length of time. Mike does not walk the dog for an hour after it has eaten. If he is short of time, he takes the dog for either a run or a shorter walk. These are temporal factors that influence the timing, length and pace of Mike's walks.

The example of occupational performance used here is Mike's twice daily walks with his dog. From this example, it is possible to see how the environment both demands Mike's performance and shapes it. Any changes in the physical, sociocultural or temporal features of the environment demand and shape corresponding changes in Mike's performance.

CONTEXT

The word *context* is sometimes used interchangeably with *environment* or *setting* but in the European conceptual framework it is given a distinct meaning. This section explores what the word means in common usage and how it has been used in the occupational therapy literature. It finishes with an explanation of the European definition of *context*.

What context means in common usage

The term *context* is often used to refer to the written word, meaning the parts immediately preceding or following a passage or word that help to determine its meaning (*Shorter Oxford English Dictionary* 2002). For example, we might talk about taking a phrase out of context when we want to indicate that its intended meaning has been changed or lost.

The other meaning of *context*, given in the *Shorter Oxford English Dictionary* (2002), is 'ambient conditions' or 'a set of circumstances'. In general use, the two meanings of the word tend to be conflated, so that ambient conditions or circumstances are seen as a context when they help to clarify or determine the meaning of an object or event. For example, 'without context, words and actions have no meaning at all' (Bateson 1979, quoted in Whiteford, Klomp and Wright-St Clair 2005, p.14).

The ICF (World Health Organization 2001) incorporates those contextual factors that impact on health, describing them as influences on functioning and disability. They include both environmental (external) factors and personal (internal) factors.

How occupational therapists use the term context

Occupational therapists use the word *context* to refer to the working environment when they want to imply that it influences how they practise, as in: 'The nature of practice also changes with the context of practice' (Ryan 1998, p.48). Sinclair (1998) used the word in this way when she wrote about the therapist's attempts to grapple with an ill-structured problem: 'To put this into a healthcare context, as the professional tries to make sense of a puzzling or interesting situation, he or she reflects on the pattern of assessment, decision-making, implementation or evaluation' (p.68). An occupational therapy textbook (Creek and Lougher 2008) includes a section, entitled 'The context of occupational therapy', with chapters on: ethics; roles and settings; the developing student practitioner, and working in a transcultural context.

Ormston (2008) was explicit about the influence of context on practice when she wrote that the *National Service Framework for Mental Health* 'continues to determine service models and standards for mental health and sets the context behind the more detailed mental health commissioning guidelines' (p.213).

The most comprehensive exploration of the meaning of the practice context for occupational therapists, to date, can be found in a book called *Occupation and Practice in Context* (Whiteford and Wright-St Clair 2005).

This edited text discusses four contexts for occupational therapy practice: the professional context; the organizational context; the sociocultural context, and the political and economic context. Within these four practice contexts, various authors have explored such concepts as theoretical contexts, international contexts, intellectual contexts and moral contexts.

Sakellariou and Pollard (2009) wrote about the contexts in which people live and perform their occupations. They observed that individuals and their contexts are often seen by occupational therapists as separate entities, but argued that:

> Context is not simply where the individual is located or occupation takes place but, rather, it can be seen as an active and vital component; individual and context are engaged in a dialectical relationship through occupation, each informing and shaping the other. (*ibid.*,p.93)

As discussed in the previous section, some occupational therapists use the words *environment* and *context* together. For example: 'considering a client's role performance in terms of its environmental context' (Bridge and Twible 1997, p.163), and 'the environmental context of activity' (Henderson 2001, p.421). Christiansen and Baum (1997, p.61) described environment as 'the context for performance' and McMillan (2006, p.259) wrote about 'the context of the environment which may facilitate or inhibit…occupations'. The latter two phrases make sense because they imply that the environment becomes a context when it is the setting for occupational performance.

Jenkins (1998) used the phrase 'lifeworld context' to refer to where a person is at a particular point in time, 'in being, not in place' (p.29), and described how the occupational therapist's focus on real-life situations 'has the effect of contextualising the client in his or her own lived-in reality' (p.30). 'The picture is one of a practice where interrelationships between practitioner and client, between client and his or her lifeworld context, between practitioner and his or her professional world context are pivotal' (p.31).

How context is understood within the conceptual framework

· ·

Context is the relationships between the environment, personal factors and events that influence the meaning of a task, activity or occupation for the performer.

· ·

This definition was constructed from two elements found in existing definitions of *context* in the occupational therapy literature:

- the relationships between the environment, personal factors and events
- influence the meaning of a task, activity or occupation for the performer.

As discussed above, the environment is the physical, sociocultural and temporal factors that demand and shape occupational performance. Personal factors are 'the attributes of the person' (World Health Organization 2001, p.11). The external environment and the individual's personal attributes interact with life events, both trivial daily experiences and major happenings, as shown in Example 11.1.

Example 11.1: Interactions between the environment, personal factors and events

John and Claire separated after nearly 20 years of marriage. There was no infidelity involved but they agreed that they no longer cared enough for each other to stay together.

This event did not entail major changes to Claire's physical or social environments. She kept the family home because their two daughters were still at secondary school, so she did not have to put time and energy into finding and setting up a new household. She continued to work full time as a teacher and to attend the local church, where she sang in the choir. There was a perception among the couple's friends that Claire was the injured party, so many of them chose to remain close to Claire and to stop seeing John. However, Claire had married young and she was not accustomed to making decisions on her own. In the evenings, she liked to unwind by discussing the events of the day with a sympathetic adult. After John moved out, she felt lonely and aggrieved, blaming him for the breakdown of their marriage. She made it plain to her daughters that she did not like them to have contact with their father. She hoped to find another partner but did not have the confidence to go to new places and meet new people.

When John moved out of the family home, he rented a house nearby so that he would be able to see his daughters frequently. He had recently moved to a new job, which he was enjoying, and he was making friends at work. At first, he felt lonely but he made overtures of friendship to his neighbours and began to receive invitations. He saw the change of living environment as an opportunity to make some positive changes to his way of life, and found it surprisingly satisfying to discover that he could build a comfortable home on his own. Once the divorce came through and the financial settlement had been agreed, he bought a small house and renovated it. He was distressed to find that neither of his daughters wanted to have regular contact, but he continued to send loving messages and presents while he waited for them to adjust to their parents' break up.

John and Claire experienced their separation and divorce in very different ways, due to the interaction between the event, their physical, sociocultural and temporal environments and their personal coping styles.

Influence is action exerted by one person or thing on another person or thing to bring about changes in conduct, development, etc. Meaning is the significance or importance that something has for a person. Interactions between the environment, personal factors and events, therefore, change the way that a performer understands what she is doing and the significance that her actions have for her. This means that a particular set of actions will be experienced differently within different contexts, even if the physical environment is unchanged, as shown in Example 11.2.

Example 11.2: How context changes the experience of occupation

After working as a volunteer in a local charity shop for four years, Fran applies for the post of manager and is appointed to work three days a week for a pro-rata salary. She continues to work as an unpaid volunteer on two other days. Fran's work includes managing the stock, maintaining the physical environment of the shop, co-ordinating the other volunteers, advertising for new stock and selling goods. She performs the same tasks on all the days when she is working in the shop.

On the days when she is being paid to work, Fran feels proud that her contribution to the shop is valued enough for her to receive a salary. On the days when she is volunteering, she feels as though she is being exploited because her work is still just as valuable but no one is paying for it. The physical environment of the shop and the tasks that Fran performs are unchanged, but the context is different on the days when her work is paid from when it is unpaid, and this changes the meaning of her occupational performance.

RELATIONSHIPS BETWEEN TERMS IN THE PLACE FOR ACTION

The three terms in the place for action cluster are close in meaning and, as identified above, may be used synonymously by occupational therapists. They all refer to the external surroundings that influence performance. *Setting* refers to the immediate surroundings in which performance takes place; *environment* can include the immediate surroundings as well as a much wider range of physical and social factors, and *context* includes both environment and personal factors.

The setting of a task, activity or occupation influences how it is performed. For example, Charlotte can cook a meal much faster and more easily in her own kitchen than in someone else's because she is familiar with where everything is kept.

Environments not only influence how occupations are performed but they demand occupational performance. For example, doing the housework is one of Charlotte's occupations. When the laundry basket in the bathroom is full, she puts a load of washing into the machine. However, if the laundry basket only has a few things in it, Charlotte does not bother doing any washing that day.

The context of a piece of performance can influence both how it is done and the meaning that it has for the performer. For example, Fred is a good chess player. When he is competing in a tournament, he takes the game very seriously and tries his best to win. He is also teaching his young nephew to play chess and when they play a game together Fred tries not to win too easily so that the boy is not discouraged. The context of the game of chess changes both how Fred performs and what the game means to him.

Shifting perspectives

Context is an abstract concept that cannot be observed, and it is the interactions between factors in a context that influence the meaning of performance, not those factors themselves. For example, if Fred's nephew was not related to him, not young, or not keen to learn chess, Fred would not take the time to teach him. It is the interaction between Fred's nephew's youth and enthusiasm that gives meaning to the occupation of teaching chess.

Setting and environment are mostly concrete and observable. For example, the kitchen is the setting for Charlotte cooking a meal, and the kitchen can be seen. The type of food that Charlotte chooses to cook is influenced by the fact that she lives in the temporal environment of the twenty-first century. We cannot directly observe the temporal influences on Charlotte's cooking but we can see the ingredients she has bought, the recipe books she owns and what she cooks; and we might know that a cook in the eighteenth century would have produced a very different meal.

Setting, environment and context all give meaning to occupational performance, so that the meaning changes as the setting, environment or context change, as shown in Example 11.3.

Example 11.3: How setting, environment and context change the meaning of performance

A local theatre company uses a church hall for their rehearsals. This setting is ideal for the purpose because the space is large enough and it is close to the theatre so that they do not have far to carry costumes and properties. For the actors and other members of the company, the church hall is not a comfortable environment because it is dusty and draughty, but they tolerate its shortcomings because it is cheap and convenient. Performances in the church hall are always rehearsals, providing a context for experimentation and repetition until the director is satisfied with the result.

The theatre where shows are performed is an old building that has been restored with charitable funding. The company are very proud of it and love performing in such an elegant environment. They feel that the Georgian architecture of the theatre provides a perfect setting for the musical comedies that they specialize in performing. Performing in a show for a paying audience feels very different from performing in a dusty rehearsal hall, and the cast always do their best in this context.

The setting in which a task or activity is performed can be seen as part of the context for that performance, as can the environment: context is always more than simply the immediate surroundings or the environment. However, setting is more than just the immediate physical environment and also includes sociocultural and temporal factors in the immediate surroundings.

Environments exist whether or not performance is taking place. For example, the kitchen is always there, even when Charlotte is not cooking in it. Setting and context are always the setting or context for a particular piece of performance. For example, the environment of a theatre can become the setting for the performance of a play, or the context for a triumphant performance by the leading lady. After the play is finished, the theatre is still an environment but it ceases to be a setting or context until the next performance.

SUMMARY

This chapter described the last cluster of terms in the European conceptual framework for occupational therapy: the place for action. The three terms used by occupational therapists to refer to where action takes place were discussed in depth: *setting*, *environment* and *context*. The chapter looked at the common usage of the terms and the ways in which they are used by occupational therapists. The European definition of each term was given, with an explanation of how the definition was constructed and what it means. The final section of the chapter explored the relationships between the three terms.

This section of the book has described the conceptual framework from the perspective of the person performing tasks, activities and occupations. The third section of the book shifts to the observer perspective, looking at how occupations, activities and tasks can be analysed, measured and used for therapeutic purposes.

REFERENCES

Bridge, C.E. and Twible, R.L. (1997) 'Clinical reasoning: informed decision making for practice.' In C. Christiansen and C. Baum (eds) *Occupational Therapy: Enabling Function and Well-being, Second Edition.* Thorofare, NJ: Slack.

Canadian Association of Occupational Therapists Health Canada (1993) *Occupational Therapy Guidelines for Client-centred Mental Health Practice.* Toronto: CAOT Publications ACE.

Christiansen, C. and Baum, C. (1997) 'Person-environment occupational performance: a conceptual model for practice.' In C. Christiansen and C. Baum (eds) *Occupational Therapy: Enabling Function and Well-being, Second Edition.* Thorofare, NJ: Slack.

Creek, J. (2008) 'The knowledge base of occupational therapy.' In J. Creek and L. Lougher (eds) *Occupational Therapy and Mental Health, Fourth Edition.* Edinburgh: Churchill Livingstone Elsevier.

Creek, J. and Lougher, L. (2008) *Occupational Therapy and Mental Health, Fourth Edition.* Edinburgh: Churchill Livingstone Elsevier.

Dunning, H. (1972) 'Environmental occupational therapy.' *American Journal of Occupational Therapy 26,* 6, 292–298.

Fougeyrollas, P. (1997) 'The influence of the social environment on the social participation of people with disabilities.' In C. Christiansen and C. Baum (eds) *Occupational Therapy: Enabling Function and Well-being, Second Edition.* Thorofare, NJ: Slack.

Hagedorn, R. (2001) *Foundations for Practice in Occupational Therapy, Third Edition.* Edinburgh: Churchill Livingstone.

Henderson, A. (2001) 'The scope of occupational science.' In R. Zemke and F. Clark (eds) *Occupational Science: The Evolving Discipline.* Philadelphia, PA: F.A. Davis.

Howe, M.C. and Briggs, A.K. (1982) 'Ecological systems model for occupational therapy.' *American Journal of Occupational Therapy 36,* 5, 322–327.

Jenkins, M. (1998) 'Shifting ground or sifting sand?' In J. Creek (ed.) *Occupational Therapy: New Perspectives.* London: Whurr.

Law, M., Cooper, B.A., Strong, S., Stewart, B., Rigby, P. and Letts, L. (1997) 'Theoretical contexts for the practice of occupational therapy.' In C. Christiansen and C. Baum (eds) *Occupational Therapy: Enabling Function and Well-being, Second Edition.* Thorofare, NJ: Slack.

Llorens, L.A. (1984) 'Changing balance: environment and individual.' *American Journal of Occupational Therapy 38,* 1, 29–34.

McMillan, I.R. (2006) 'Assumptions underpinning a biomechanical frame of reference in occupational therapy.' In E.A.S. Duncan (ed.) *Foundations for Practice in Occupational Therapy, Fourth Edition.* Edinburgh: Elsevier Churchill Livingstone.

Mosey, A.C. (1986) *Psychosocial Components of Occupational Therapy.* New York: Raven Press.

Ormston, C. (2008) 'Roles and settings.' In J. Creek and L. Lougher (eds) *Occupational Therapy and Mental Health, Fourth Edition.* Edinburgh: Churchill Livingstone Elsevier.

Polgar, J.M. and Landry, J.E. (2004) 'Occupations as means for individual and group participation in life.' In C.H. Christiansen and E.A. Townsend (eds) *Introduction to Occupation: The Art and Science of Living.* Upper Saddle River, NJ: Prentice Hall.

Reed, K.L. and Sanderson, S.N. (1992) *Concepts of Occupational Therapy, Third Edition.* Baltimore, MD: Williams & Wilkins.

Ryan, S. (1998) 'Influences that shape our reasoning.' In J. Creek (ed.) *Occupational Therapy: New Perspectives.* London: Whurr.

Sakellariou, D. and Pollard, N. (2009) 'Political challenges of holism: heteroglossia and the (im)possibility of holism.' In N. Pollard, D. Sakellariou and F. Kronenberg (eds) *A Political Practice of Occupational Therapy.* Edinburgh: Churchill Livingstone Elsevier.

Sinclair, K. (1998) 'Reflective practice in health care.' In J. Creek (ed.) *Occupational Therapy: New Perspectives.* London: Whurr.

Shorter Oxford English Dictionary, Fifth Edition (2002) Oxford: Oxford University Press.

Wilcock, A.A. (1998) *An Occupational Perspective of Health.* Thorofare, NJ: Slack.

Whiteford, G., Klomp, N. and Wright-St Clair, V. (2005) 'Complexity theory: understanding occupation, practice and context.' In G. Whiteford and V. Wright-St Clair (eds) *Occupation and Practice in Context.* Sydney: Elsevier Churchill Livingstone.

Whiteford, G. and Wright-St Clair, V. (2005) *Occupation and Practice in Context.* Sydney: Elsevier Churchill Livingstone.

World Health Organization (1986) *Ottawa Charter for Health Promotion.* Geneva: World health Organization

World Health Organization (2001) *ICF: International Classification of Functioning, Disability and Health.* Geneva: World Health Organization.

SECTION 3

THE OBSERVER'S PERSPECTIVE

Chapter 12: Understanding Action

Chapter 13: Measuring Action

Chapter 14: Facilitating Action

Section 2 of the book explored the terms in the conceptual framework from the perspective of the person performing occupations and activities. The three chapters in Section 3 consider occupation from the perspective of the observer. The terms defined in Chapters 12 and 13 are *task analysis, activity analysis, occupational mapping, assessment* and *evaluation*. These terms represent five of the core skills of the occupational therapist. Chapter 14 describes how these skills are applied in practice.

Throughout occupational therapy intervention, the therapist is the observer of the client's performance, seeking to understand, measure and facilitate his occupations and activities. This section of the book explains how the European conceptual framework can be used to guide occupational therapy practice.

CHAPTER 12

UNDERSTANDING ACTION

INTRODUCTION

In order to be able to use activity as a therapeutic medium, the occupational therapist has to achieve a deep understanding of what people do, how they do it and why they do it. This understanding comes from knowing the parameters of occupation, which are represented by the terms in the European conceptual framework, and from recognizing that these parameters are not context-free and static but constantly change in relation to each other and in response to circumstances. The occupational therapist, therefore, studies both occupations and the performance of occupations.

Occupational therapists have developed many theories of occupation, such as occupational behaviour (Reilly 1969), occupational genesis (Breines 1995) and occupational deprivation (Wilcock 1998). The abstract, acontextual knowledge embodied in these theories is translated into practical knowledge of particular occupations, and of the pattern and meaning that occupations have for each individual, through exercising the skills of *task analysis, activity analysis* and *occupational mapping.*

Allen (1985, p.79) pointed out that 'it is difficult to separate the person doing the task from the task itself; occupational therapists have trouble with this distinction'. This chapter will try to make clear the distinction by identifying how we can know those aspects of occupation that exist independent of the performer, which Allen calls the task. Aspects of individual performance are explored in the section of this chapter on *occupational mapping*, which discusses how we can explore a person's occupations, but are addressed more fully in Chapter 13, which covers *assessment* and *evaluation*.

The ways in which we can understand both the task and the person doing the task are described from the perspective of the therapist as observer of the client's performance.

How the chapter is organized

This chapter explores the meaning of three core occupational therapy concepts: *task analysis, activity analysis* and *occupational mapping*. The term *occupational mapping* was selected, rather than *occupational analysis*, because it better describes the collaborative process by which the client and therapist move towards recognition and understanding of the individual's unique pattern of occupations.

The chapter begins with an exploration of the meaning of *analysis* in general usage. It reviews how occupational therapists use the term *task analysis* and presents the European definition, with an explanation of how it was constructed. The chapter then reviews how occupational therapists use the term *activity analysis* and presents the European definition, with an explanation of how it was constructed. The term *occupational mapping* was adopted from a European Network of Occupational Therapy in Higher Education (ENOTHE) publication on activity analysis and defined by the terminology group. Its meaning and use are discussed here.

TASK ANALYSIS AND ACTIVITY ANALYSIS

The concepts of *task analysis* and *activity analysis* are important to occupational therapists, and both terms are widely used in the literature. However, there is some confusion between the two concepts, which this chapter will try to resolve. Both terms refer to specialized aspects of the occupational therapist's work and are not found in general usage.

What analysis means in common usage

Analysis is both a way of observing and a way of thinking. *Analysis* is defined as 'the resolution or breaking up of something complex into its various simple elements; the exact determination of the elements or components of something complex' (*Shorter Oxford English Dictionary* 2002). To *analyse* something is to ascertain its elements or to examine minutely its constitution (*Shorter Oxford English Dictionary* 2002). For example, a manager might analyse the performance of his department in order to work out how its operation could be made more efficient. To do this, he identifies all the elements that constitute the working of the department and what they contribute to the process.

The word *analysis* is more commonly used in the context of work than other areas of daily life. For example, analysis is likely to be an important aspect of the work of a scientist but it is unlikely to be seen as part of the occupation of parenting.

Psychoanalysis is a method of treatment for mental health problems, originated by Freud, which involves bringing into consciousness those unconscious anxieties and conflicts that are creating problems.

How occupational therapists use the term task analysis

Various definitions of *task analysis* can be found in the occupational therapy literature, for example:

- discovering the sequence of steps or tasks that make up an activity (Creek and Lougher 2008, p.583)

- examining an activity to identify the sequence of steps or tasks that constitute the activity (Creek 2003, p.60)

- breaking down the task into subtasks and analysing the general categories of motor, cognitive or interactive skills required at each stage or at a particular stage (Hagedorn 2001, p.42)

- the examination and ordering of the tasks that comprise an activity, rather than the activity as a whole...defining and grading the sequential steps that comprise the given tasks of an activity (Fidler 1999, p.48).

It can be seen from these definitions that some occupational therapists see task analysis as simply identifying the sequence of tasks that make up an activity while others include identification of the components of the task, such as the skills required for its performance: 'some task analyses focus on task content; others, on task procedures' (Allen 1985, p.9).

Hagedorn (2000, p.191) pointed out that 'task analysis is a reductive, atomistic, analytical process which is most applicable to high visibility performance which is relatively simple, structured and sequenced'. She wrote that task analysis consists of both sequence analysis (identifying the sequence of tasks in an activity) and content analysis (identifying the purpose, participants, practical requirements, location and standards of the activity).

Task analysis is sometimes seen as one part of activity analysis, as in this definition: activity analysis is 'a process of dissecting an activity into its component parts and task sequence' (Creek 2003, p.49). In practice, an occupational therapist is likely to identify the task sequence of an activity before examining the components of each task. This is because different tasks may make very different demands on the performer, as shown in Example 12.1.

Example 12.1: An activity comprising a sequence of varied tasks

Joan Smith's mother has been admitted to hospital and Joan wants to visit her. Together, the occupational therapist and Joan go through the sequence of tasks that she must accomplish in order to visit her mother. The first task is to find out which ward her mother is in and when the visiting times are: to get this information she telephones the hospital. The next task is to find out which bus goes from Joan's house to the hospital: to do this, she uses a search tool on the internet. The third task is to catch the right bus at the right time, by walking from her house to the bus stop. Joan then has to perform three further tasks: to sit on the bus until it arrives at the right stop; to get off, and to walk to the right ward in the hospital.

Creek and Bullock (2008) suggested that there are four reasons for carrying out a task analysis:

1. to assist in selecting an appropriate method for teaching an activity

2. to select an appropriate activity to meet a therapeutic aim

3. to adapt an activity by changing or eliminating a step

4. to identify the precise action the individual is having difficulty performing.

Any one step in the first level of task analysis can be analysed into a further series of tasks. In Example 12.1, the first step for Joan in visiting her mother is finding out which ward her mother has been admitted to, but there is a sequence of smaller steps involved in this task, as shown in Example 12.2. The process of breaking steps into sequences of smaller steps can be carried out to the point where the task does not entail a sequence of actions but is a single movement.

Example 12.2: Analysing a step into a further series of tasks

The sequence of tasks involved in finding out the ward to which Joan Smith's mother has been admitted is as follows:

1. Locate the telephone.

2. Find the telephone number of the hospital.

3. Telephone the hospital.

4. Ask the receptionist which ward Mrs Smith has been admitted to.

5. Make a note of the ward.

6. Ask the receptionist to transfer the telephone call to the ward.

7. Wait until the call is answered on the ward.

8. Check with ward staff that Mrs Smith is a patient on the ward.

9. Ask how she is.

10. Check family visiting times with the ward staff.

11. Make a note of the visiting times.

12. Ask the ward staff to give Mrs Smith a message.

13. Thank the ward staff.

14. Terminate the telephone call.

Depending on the purpose of the task analysis, it may be carried out in more or less detail. Example 12.3 shows how an occupational therapist used task analysis to identify which step of an activity the client found difficult, then analysed that step into its subtasks in order to select an appropriate teaching method.

Example 12.3: The use of task analysis in selecting an appropriate teaching method

An occupational therapist was working with a young woman, Susan, who had a mild learning disability and some hearing impairment. Susan wanted to learn how to travel independently from her home to the social centre she attended on three days a week. The occupational therapist analysed the journey into three tasks: walking to the bus stop; catching a bus to the road where the centre was located, and walking from the bus stop to the centre.

Susan already knew how to use a bus, including identifying which one to take, and she quickly learned to get off at the right stop, which was just outside the social centre. The task that she found most difficult was walking from her house to the stop where she would catch the bus, because this involved a longer walk and crossing a busy road. The therapist analysed the task of walking to the bus stop into a series of six subtasks: leaving the house; walking to the next intersection;

crossing the road; continuing to the end of the street; turning left onto the high street, and walking along the high street to the bus stop.

In order to teach Susan how to get to the bus stop, the therapist used backward chaining. She accompanied Susan for the first five tasks, allowing her to complete the sixth task, walking along the high street to the bus stop, by herself. When Susan was confident in completing this task by herself, the therapist accompanied her for the first four tasks, allowing her to complete the last two tasks by herself. This process was continued until Susan felt confident that she could walk to the bus stop independently.

The European definition of task analysis

The European definition of *analysis* was constructed from elements found in existing definitions of the term:

· ·

Analysis is breaking up something into its component parts.

· ·

Within the European conceptual framework, the word *task* is given two definitions (see Chapters 4 and 10):

1. A series of structured steps (actions and/or thoughts) intended to accomplish the performance of an activity.

2. A series of structured steps (actions and/or thoughts) intended to accomplish the performance of a piece of work the individual is expected to do.

The first of these definitions is the one relevant to the concept of task analysis, so that *task analysis* means breaking up an activity into a series of structured steps (actions and/or thoughts) intended to accomplish its performance. This definition has been simplified to become:

· ·

Task analysis is breaking up an activity into its task sequence.

· ·

Through task analysis, the observer (therapist) identifies the sequence of tasks that is intended to accomplish the performance of an activity. This sequence of tasks is identified independent of a specific context: that is, the therapist analyses the activity itself, not the performance of a person doing the activity. This means that the analysis will not be relevant to everyone, since different people will perform the same activity in different ways. The same activity may be accomplished through a different sequence of tasks, either by different people or by the same person on different occasions, as shown in Example 12.4. What is most important is not the sequence of tasks itself but that it accomplishes the performance of the activity. This flexibility of tasks and task sequence is one of the features of activity that makes possible activity adaptation.

Example 12.4: Different task sequences in the performance of the same activity

During an energy conservation group for people with chronic obstructive pulmonary disease, the topic of packing a suitcase was raised. One woman said that she put the suitcase open on a spare bed and placed items in it over the course of several days, as they came to hand. On the day before departure, she took out all the contents of the case and laid them on the bed, before repacking them neatly. A man in the group said that he always made a list of what to pack. When he was more active, he used to pack everything on the list the night before departure. Now that he has less energy, he takes a few days to pack, starting with the heavier items, such as shoes, and finishing with the lighter objects, such as shirts.

The particular tasks selected to accomplish an activity, and the sequence in which they are performed, are influenced by such factors as culture, personal preference, environment and context. For example, an occupational therapist working in a multicultural community will probably find that her clients have a range of approaches to managing their personal hygiene. They all accomplish the activity of washing but the task sequence and the tasks themselves might vary widely.

How occupational therapists use the term activity analysis

Like task analysis, activity analysis is considered to be a core skill of the occupational therapist. It is one of the tools that enable the therapist to use the activities of everyday life as therapeutic media. However, there are many different understandings of activity analysis, some of which are explored here.

A historical analysis of the origins and evolution of the use of activity analysis by occupational therapists in America led to the conclusion that 'the term *activity analysis* and the methodology for breaking down and examining tasks scientifically...were borrowed from industry during World War I' (Creighton 1992, p.45). Activity analysis was used to identify the demands of the activity and the ways in which it could be adapted so that people with disabilities would be able to perform it.

Although activity analysis is widely accepted as a central component of occupational therapy practice, it is understood in many different ways, as shown by the following selection of definitions:

- a process of dissecting an activity into its component parts and task sequence in order to identify its inherent properties and the skills required for its performance, thus allowing the therapist to evaluate its therapeutic potential (Creek 2003, p.49)

- the thought processes practitioners use when thinking about activities in general (Crepeau 2003, p.190)

- dissection of an activity into its component tasks and the evaluation of therapeutic potential and relevance to the treatment plan; investigating the objective or subjective performance components (Hagedorn 2001, p.160)

- a process that assesses the elements or characteristics of an activity for the purpose of identifying and defining the dimensions of its performance requirements and its social and cultural significance and meanings (Fidler 1999, p.4)

- the process of examining an activity to distinguish its component parts (Mosey 1986, p.12).

Two of these definitions include identification of the tasks that constitute the activity, four include identification of its component parts and two include identification of performance demands. The performance demands of an activity are the skills required for its performance, such as mobility or concentration. Other components include the actual and symbolic meanings of an activity and its social and cultural purpose and value (Creek and Bullock 2008). Creek described the identification of the performance demands of an activity as basic activity analysis and identification of other components as extended activity analysis, which requires the exercise of reflection in addition to analysis (Creek 2007a; Creek and Bullock 2008).

Activity analysis can be used to discover all the component parts of an activity that come within the domain of the occupational therapist, or it can focus on the components that are relevant to the particular theory or frame of reference that the therapist is using (Creek and Bullock 2008).

For example, Fidler and Fidler (1963, p.75) designed a format to be used within an object relations frame of reference, which focused on 'the basic and fundamental psychodynamic characteristics of a given activity', such as the resistiveness of materials, opportunities to express feelings freely and the symbols inherent in methods of procedure, materials, equipment and end product.

The term job analysis has recently been used in the occupational therapy literature (Joss 2007) in relation to work rehabilitation. Job analysis is defined as 'a systematic approach to identify and describe the demands that a job places on a worker' (p.301). This is a narrower conceptualization of analysis than that used in the European definition of activity analysis, which is given below.

The European definition of activity analysis

The European definition of *activity analysis* was constructed from the definitions of *analysis* and *activity performance*. As described above, *analysis* means breaking up something into its component parts. *Activity analysis* is the process of breaking up *activity performance* into its component parts. *Activity performance* is defined as choosing, organizing and carrying out activities in interaction with the environment. From these definitions we can see that:

· ·

Activity analysis is breaking up an activity into the components that influence how it is chosen, organized and carried out in interaction with the environment.

· ·

The process of activity analysis focuses on the activity, not on the person doing the activity:

> The purpose of an activity analysis is to arrive at an understanding of the activity's inherent qualities and characteristics, its meaning in and of itself, irrespective of a performer. Only after such an analysis has been made can one begin to discern the probable impact of an activity on an individual or group. (Fidler 1999, p.47)

The components of activity, that influence how it is chosen, organized and carried out in interaction with the environment, are represented by the terms in the European conceptual framework, as summarized in Box 12.1.

Box 12.1: The components of activity

- Occupation

- Activity

- Task (a piece of work that the individual is expected to do)

- Task (steps in the performance of an activity)

- Habit

- Routine

- Task performance

- Activity performance

- Occupational performance

- Occupational performance areas

- Occupational performance components (abilities and skills)

- Function (occupational performance components and the capacity to use them)

- Motivation

- Volition

- Engagement

- Context

- Environment (physical, sociocultural and temporal)

- Setting

- Participation

- Role

- Autonomy

- Dependence, independence and interdependence

Analysis of a particular activity does not necessarily take into account all these components: activity analysis is always done for a purpose and will focus on different aspects of the activity depending on that purpose. For example, if the occupational therapist is selecting activities to use with a group of people who have chronic depression, she may focus on aspects of the activity that could influence motivation, volition, engagement, participation, autonomy and interdependence. If she is choosing an activity to help someone develop hand function following a stroke, she may focus on task performance, activity performance, occupational performance components, context, setting, motivation, volition and engagement.

When thinking about aspects of activity that might promote or inhibit the client's engagement (Creek 2007a), the occupational therapist is aware that such factors are not universal: a factor that attracts one person may repel another person, as shown in Example 12.5.

Example 12.5: A factor that can promote or inhibit engagement in activity

An occupational therapist working in a social services day centre ran a weekly arts and crafts group for women experiencing long-term, severe mental health problems. After a few months, one of the women suggested that they should visit the local art gallery where they could have a cup of coffee, see an exhibition and browse in the craft shop. Everyone agreed that this was a good idea and that they would meet at the gallery.

On the day of the gallery visit, the therapist was surprised to find that only about a third of the group members turned up. Subsequently, during individual sessions, she asked what people had felt about the activity. The women who had visited the art gallery said that they liked going somewhere public, with the support of the therapist and the group, rather than just staying in the day centre. The women who did not go to the art gallery said that they did not feel comfortable going into a public place with a group of fellow patients.

For some of the patients, the social context of the activity (going to a public place with fellow group members) felt comfortable and supportive. For others, it felt inappropriate and uncomfortable.

When the occupational therapist has identified the components of an activity, she has also to think about how they relate to each other. As described in Chapter 3, relationships between concepts in the European conceptual framework are not fixed but become stronger or weaker in different contexts, as illustrated by Example 12.6.

Example 12.6: How new clusters of terms form during specific activities

A group of four young men with moderate learning disabilities lived in a small, purpose-built residential unit. They all had serious communication difficulties and exhibited a range of self-injurious behaviours, such as head banging. The psychiatrist asked the occupational therapist if she could find a way of helping them to develop more effective strategies for managing their feelings, with the aim of reducing incidents of self-harm.

The therapist decided to run a non-verbal supportive psychotherapy group to enable the men to identify and express how they were feeling. She chose listening to music as the medium for the first sessions, reasoning that this activity would draw on and develop the participants' personal requisites for action, which are: *occupational performance components* (psychosocial and affective abilities and skills); *ability* (to see, to hear, to sit, to experience emotion); *skill* (to sit still, to pay attention, to listen, to take turns, to communicate); *function 1* (sight, hearing, affect), and *function 2* (participation in the music group).

During the first session, it became apparent that group members were not accustomed to sitting still and listening to music for an extended period of time; all of them had left the room by the end of the session. The therapist had to adapt the group so that everyone would remain for the full hour in order to benefit from the group. At the beginning of the next session, she told participants that everyone who was in the room at the end would be given tea and biscuits. The key components of this activity were: *motivation* (desire for tea and biscuits); *autonomy* (freedom to choose to stay or to leave the group), and *task 2* (requirement to be in the room at the end of the session).

After several sessions, the therapist found that group members left the room less frequently and were more likely to come back. They sat still for longer and were quieter while the music was playing. Some of them responded when the therapist asked them questions about the music. At this stage of the group, the key components of the activity became those in the cluster of personal requisites for action, plus three additional components: *routine* (established time for listening to music); *motivation* (desire for tea and biscuits, desire to listen to music), and *participation* (involvement in the music group).

To analyse something is to break it into its component parts but the occupational therapist always thinks about how those parts fit together, as shown in Example 12.6. The next section looks at how the therapist and client work through these processes together during *occupational mapping*.

OCCUPATIONAL MAPPING

As explained in the introduction, the term *occupational mapping* was selected, rather than *occupational analysis*, to represent the process by which the occupational therapist works with the client to identify and understand the nature, range and balance of occupations in his life. Mapping the client's occupations is important because change often depends on the client reaching an understanding of his own occupations, rather than this knowledge being held by the occupational therapist.

What mapping means in common usage

To map means to 'establish the relative positions, or the spatial relations or distribution, of [an object or its components]' (*Shorter Oxford English Dictionary* 2002). Mapping something means establishing its position in relation to other things, including the spatial relationship and distribution. For example, mapping the bird population of the North York Moors National Park means establishing what birds can be found there, how many there are of each species and where they can be found in relation to each other and to features of the physical environment.

How occupational therapists use the term occupational mapping

The term *occupational mapping* was coined by members of the ENOTHE activity analysis project working group to refer to how occupational therapists approach the task of understanding an individual's occupations (Morel-Bracq *et al.* 2008). Occupational mapping is described as a collaborative process between the therapist, the client and the social environment by which participants attempt to capture the complexity of the individual's occupations within a particular context.

In contrast to activity analysis, which focuses on the activity, occupational mapping focuses on the person performing the activity: on his experience of occupation and performance. Occupational mapping, therefore, requires the person to reflect on his own performance and values. This is a subjective process, which the therapist attempts to facilitate in the client so that he achieves a deeper understanding of his occupations, 'thus increasing [his] responsibility, choice, autonomy and control' (Creek 2003, p.8).

The European definition of occupational mapping

The European definition of occupational mapping was constructed from descriptions given in the ENOTHE publication, *Teaching and Learning: Activity Analysis and Occupational Mapping* (Morel-Bracq *et al.* 2008):

••

Occupational mapping is a collaborative process between the therapist and client through which the person's subjective experience of occupation can be explored.

••

The concept of occupational mapping is similar to Creek's extended activity analysis, which seeks to elicit the meaning that an activity has for the individual, how it might tap into his motivation, the effect it has on his identity and the opportunities it brings for learning and personal growth (Creek and Bullock 2008).

The therapist is always the observer of the client's performance, therefore occupational mapping has to be a collaborative process. If the therapist wants to work in a client-centred way, she needs to understand the client's perspective on what he is doing and to respond flexibly when his perceptions change. Part of the art of therapy is being able to recognize when the client's perspective shifts and to adjust the intervention accordingly, as illustrated in Example 12.7.

Example 12.7: Recognizing when the client's perspective shifts

Mr Plummer was referred to the crisis intervention team with severe depression after being made redundant when his job was contracted out to a company in India. In occupational therapy terms, he had lost one of his main occupations. One of the aims of the team was to encourage him to look for alternative work (a new occupation), but he refused to consider this. The occupational therapist recognized that Mr Plummer was grieving for his lost occupation, and that grieving was the occupation in which he needed to engage at the present time.

The therapist spent some weeks helping Mr Plummer to work through his feelings. Eventually, he felt ready to move forward and the therapist then supported him in exploring employment options. The therapist was able to observe the moment at which her client was ready to replace the occupation of grieving with the occupation of looking for work.

Different types of thinking are required during the process of occupational mapping, as the therapist and client together seek to understand the client's subjective experience. These types of thinking include analysis, reflection, problem sensing, evaluation and judgement (Creek 2007b; Sinclair 2007). The therapist's task is to support the client in thinking about his occupations, using her knowledge of occupation as a guide. This process is illustrated in Example 12.8.

Example 12.8: Supporting the client in thinking about his occupations

Mrs Potts was referred to the occupational therapist for advice on time-structuring, as part of a strategy to control her drinking. During the initial interview, it emerged that Mrs Potts had begun drinking when her husband left her for a younger woman. She then lost her job as a teaching assistant because her cognitive functioning was impaired by excessive alcohol consumption. At the time of referral, drinking was her main occupation, taking up a large part of her time.

Over a period of several weeks, the therapist worked with Mrs Potts to map the range of occupations that she had engaged in before the breakdown of her marriage. The therapist supported Mrs Potts in identifying which occupations were no longer available to her and which ones she could still engage in if she controlled her drinking. Mrs Potts was able to reflect on what the loss of two major occupations (marriage and employment) meant to her in terms of loss of identity, empty time, financial hardship and so on. She then began to think about which of her present occupations might be expanded to meet her needs and what new occupations she could seek.

SUMMARY

This chapter, the first one to address the perspective of the therapist as observer of the client's performance, has examined the skills that occupational therapists use to reach an understanding of occupation and activity. These skills are *task analysis, activity analysis* and *occupational mapping.*

Through task analysis and activity analysis, the occupational therapist is able to identify the task sequence and components of an activity, including its performance demands and therapeutic potential. These skills allow the therapist to select, synthesize and adapt activities for individual clients and for particular purposes.

By employing occupational mapping, in collaboration with the client, the occupational therapist is able to understand the person's experience of occupation, including 'the nature, balance, pattern and context of occupations in [his] life' (Creek 2003, p.31). This skill enables the occupational therapist to select, synthesize or adapt activities to engage the active participation of the client in the therapeutic process.

Chapter 13, which is also written from the observer perspective, explores the terms that refer to how the occupational therapist comes to understand the occupational performance of the client: *assessment* and *evaluation.*

REFERENCES

Allen, C.K. (1985) *Occupational Therapy for Psychiatric Diseases: Measurement and Management of Cognitive Disabilities.* Boston, MA: Little Brown and Company.

Breines, E.B. (1995) *Occupational Therapy Activities from Clay to Computers: Theory and Practice.* Philadelphia, PA: F.A. Davis.

Creek, J. (2003) *Occupational Therapy Defined as a Complex Intervention.* London: College of Occupational Therapists.

Creek, J. (2007a) 'Engaging the reluctant client.' In J. Creek and A. Lawson-Porter (eds) *Contemporary Issues in Occupational Therapy: Reasoning and Reflection.* Chichester: Wiley.

Creek, J. (2007b) 'The thinking therapist.' In J. Creek and A. Lawson-Porter (eds) *Contemporary Issues in Occupational Therapy: Reasoning and Reflection.* Chichester: Wiley.

Creek, J. and Bullock, A. (2008) 'Planning and implementation.' In J. Creek and L. Lougher (eds) *Occupational Therapy and Mental Health, Fourth Edition.* Edinburgh: Churchill Livingstone Elsevier.

Creek, J. and Lougher, L. (2008) *Occupational Therapy and Mental Health, Fourth Edition.* Edinburgh: Churchill Livingstone Elsevier.

Creighton, C. (1992) 'The origin and evolution of activity analysis.' *American Journal of Occupational Therapy 46,* 1, 45–48.

Crepeau, E.B. (2003) 'Analyzing occupation and activity: a way of thinking about occupational performance.' In E.B. Crepeau, E.S. Cohn and B.A.B. Schell (eds) *Willard and Spackman's Occupational Therapy, Tenth Edition.* Philadelphia, PA: Lippincott Williams & Wilkins.

Fidler, G.S. (1999) 'Deciphering the message: the activity analysis.' In G.S. Fidler and B.P. Velde *Activities: Reality and Symbol.* Thorofare, NJ: Slack.

Fidler, G.S. and Fidler, J.W. (1963) *Occupational Therapy: A Communication Process in Psychiatry.* New York: Macmillan.

Hagedorn, R. (2000) *Tools for Practice in Occupational Therapy: A Structured Approach to Core Skills and Processes.* Edinburgh: Churchill Livingstone.

Hagedorn, R. (2001) *Foundations for Practice in Occupational Therapy, Third Edition.* Edinburgh: Churchill Livingstone.

Joss, M. (2007) 'The importance of job analysis in occupational therapy.' *British Journal of Occupational Therapy 70,* 7, 301–303.

Morel-Bracq, M., Burgess-Morris, K., Cirtautas, A., Market, M., May, G. and Randlov, B. (2008) *Teaching and Learning: Activity Analysis and Occupational Mapping.* Amsterdam: ENOTHE.

Mosey, A.C. (1986) *Psychosocial Components of Occupational Therapy.* New York: Raven Press.

Reilly, M. (1969) 'The educational process.' *American Journal of Occupational Therapy 23,* 4, 299–307.

Shorter Oxford English Dictionary, Fifth Edition (2002) Oxford: Clarendon Press.

Sinclair, K. (2007) 'Exploring the facets of clinical reasoning.' In J. Creek and A. Lawson-Porter (eds) *Contemporary Issues in Occupational Therapy: Reasoning and Reflection.* Chichester: Wiley.

Wilcock, A.A. (1998) *An Occupational Perspective of Health.* Thorofare, NJ: Slack.

MEASURING ACTION

INTRODUCTION

Chapter 12 described how occupational therapists use the skills of *task analysis, activity analysis* and *occupational mapping* to reach an understanding of the components, constitution and organization of occupations. This understanding is a prerequisite for occupational therapy intervention: the therapist has to know the parameters of occupation in order to be able to assess the client's occupational performance and to use activities as therapeutic media.

In addition to understanding the features of occupation, the therapist has to be able to judge the occupational performance of individuals, groups and communities in order to identify areas of strength and weakness. The skills that the occupational therapist uses when studying occupational performance are *assessment* and *evaluation*.

Assessment may focus on the client's overall occupational performance or on any aspect of performance, including performance components and environments. The European conceptual framework provides a structure for assessing the occupational performance of individuals and groups by highlighting all the factors that influence and shape performance.

How the chapter is organized

This chapter provides a detailed examination of the concepts of *assessment* and *evaluation*. It begins with an exploration of the meaning of *assessment* in general usage, reviews how occupational therapists use the term and presents the European definition, with an explanation of how it was constructed. The chapter then looks at the meaning of evaluation in general usage, reviews how occupational therapists use the term and presents the European definition, with an explanation of how it was constructed. A case study is used throughout the chapter to illustrate how the occupational therapist organizes and carries out the process of assessment and evaluation with a client who has a long-term health condition.

ASSESSMENT

Assessment is one of the core skills of the occupational therapist (Creek 2003) and an integral part of any occupational therapy intervention. The therapist carries out a range of assessments, at different stages of the intervention, from the initial screening assessment to the final assessment of outcomes.

What the term assessment means in common usage

The term *assessment* is commonly used to refer to the estimation or measurement of various qualities, such as value, size or extent. For example, an estate agent carries out an assessment of the condition and value of a property before recommending a market price for it. Or a person talks about making a rough assessment of his projected income and outgoings for the year before deciding what type of holiday he will be able to afford. Assessment is an essential component of all educational programmes, from primary through to postgraduate study. Occupational therapy students experience a range of assessments throughout their programme, including coursework, examinations and practice placement assessment.

In everyday life, the terms assessment and evaluation are often used interchangeably. Indeed, the *Shorter Oxford English Dictionary* (2002) defines *assessment* as 'evaluation, estimation' and defines *evaluation* as 'assessment of worth'.

How occupational therapists use the term assessment

In the United Kingdom, the term *assessment* means 'the process of collecting accurate and relevant information about the client in order to set baselines and to monitor and measure the outcomes of therapy' (Creek 2003, p.50). Some writers use the term *evaluation* rather than *assessment* to refer to this process (Mosey 1986; Neistadt 1998).

The process of assessment is an integral part of the broader process of therapeutic intervention. Assessment includes collecting information relevant to the decision-making process, interpreting that information to enable clinical decision making and evaluating the outcomes of interventions (Laver Fawcett 2007).

A textbook from the mid-twentieth century (Macdonald 1976) cautioned that the purpose of assessment must always be clearly established: 'Assessment of the patient is not an end in itself and careful consideration must be given to the reasons for doing it' (p.34). This caution was echoed 30 years later: 'assessment should be recognized as a means to an end – identification of the problem, definition of a starting point for intervention, measurement of progress and evaluation of the outcome' (Duncan 2006, pp.50–51).

In these latter two definitions, evaluation is included as part of the assessment process: the evaluation of the outcomes of intervention. The concept of outcome measurement is discussed in more detail later in this chapter.

The *initial assessment* takes place at an early stage of intervention and provides information that can be used to identify problems and needs and to set goals for intervention. It has been defined as 'the art of defining the problem to be tackled or identifying the goal to be achieved' (Creek and Bullock 2008, p.83). *Ongoing assessment* is an integral part of the process of intervention which enables the therapist and client to monitor the progress of the intervention so that it can be modified, if necessary. The *final assessment* is carried out at a late stage of the intervention and demonstrates whether or not the planned goals have been met and what other changes have taken place during the course of the intervention.

Assessment of the client's occupational performance is carried out by the occupational therapist in collaboration with the client. The therapist decides what is to be assessed and selects appropriate measurement tools, but 'the effectiveness of the entire process will be enhanced...if the client understands the key issues of this working relationship' (Sumsion 1999, p.18).

Occupational therapists may use specific types of assessment, such as functional assessment and environmental assessment. Functional assessment, sometimes called functional analysis, is:

> part of the assessment process that looks at how the individual manages the normal range of daily life activities, a wide spectrum assessment that allows the therapist and client to identify the client's strengths,

problems, sociocultural environment and personal view of life. (Creek and Lougher 2008, p.581)

Mattingly, the anthropologist who carried out the American occupational therapy clinical reasoning study, described the breadth of the occupational therapy functional assessment:

> The functional assessment, which is the occupational therapy equivalent of the doctor's diagnosis, generally requires that the therapist go beyond gathering information and assessing the patient's physiological condition. It requires that the therapist pay some attention to the patient's unique life history and to how the patient sees and understands her or his condition. (Mattingly 1994, pp.74–75)

Environmental assessment, sometimes called environmental analysis, is the 'observation of features in the physical or social environment and interpretation of their significance for client performance or therapy' (Hagedorn 2001, p.161).

The European understanding of the term assessment

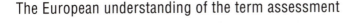

Assessment is a process of collecting, analysing and interpreting information about people's functions and environments, using observation, testing and measurement, in order to make intervention decisions and to monitor changes.

This definition was constructed from ten elements found in existing definitions of *assessment* in the occupational therapy literature:

- a process
- collecting information
- analysing information
- interpreting information
- about people's functions and environments
- using observation
- using testing
- using measurement

- in order to make intervention decisions

- in order to monitor changes.

A process is 'a continuous series of actions, events or changes' (*Shorter Oxford English Dictionary* 2002). The actions that make up the process of assessment are collecting, analysing and interpreting information. These actions do not occur only once, or in a predictable sequence, but form a continuous series in which collection, analysis and interpretation may be repeated as many times as necessary. Example 13.1 illustrates the iterative process of assessment with someone who has a chronic health condition.

To collect is 'to obtain or seek out' (*Shorter Oxford English Dictionary* 2002). To analyse something is to examine it critically in order to bring out the essential elements (*ibid.*). To *interpret* is to explain to oneself or to obtain significant information from something (*ibid.*). The occupational therapist seeks out relevant information about the client, examines it critically in order to identify the essential points and seeks to explain its significance to the occupational therapy intervention.

The information which the occupational therapist seeks is about people's functions (capacity to use occupational performance components to carry out a task, activity or occupation) and their environments (external factors that demand and shape occupational performance). It is the interaction between the individual's functions and environments that determines occupational performance.

Information about people's functions and environments may be obtained in various ways:

- Observation is 'the careful watching or noting of an object or phenomenon' (*Shorter Oxford English Dictionary 2002*).

- Testing means subjecting something to critical examination or trial (*ibid.*).

- To measure is 'to ascertain or determine the spatial magnitude or quantity of something' and measurement is 'an act of measuring' (*ibid.*).

The occupational therapist collects information about people's functions and environments in order to make intervention decisions and monitor changes, as shown in Example 13.1.

Example 13.1: The process of assessment

John is a married man in his mid-forties with a long-term health condition: chronic systemic sarcoidosis. Sarcoidosis is a granulomatous disease of unknown aetiology, which is characterized in its chronic form by progressive breathlessness. John also experiences recurrent episodes of moderate depression.

John is referred to the occupational therapist for advice on energy conservation, as part of an eight-week pulmonary rehabilitation programme. At their initial meeting, the therapist asks John to fill in a form showing the activities he does during a typical day, in order to produce an activity profile. John's lung function is then tested and the therapist notes that it is better than might have been predicted from his low levels of activity. The therapist gives John both verbal and written advice on how to carry out his daily activities more efficiently.

At the second appointment, the occupational therapist asks John to produce another activity profile, and reviews with him whether the energy conservation advice has made any difference to what he is able to do during a typical day. John's occupational performance has already improved and he expresses satisfaction with the advice he has been given. The therapist continues to monitor his function and progress during the remainder of the pulmonary rehabilitation programme.

Two years later, John is again referred by his GP for pulmonary rehabilitation following an acute episode of sarcoidosis. The therapist asks him to produce an activity profile and tests his lung function. John's lung function is only slightly reduced but his activity levels are much lower. The therapist observes that he is slightly unkempt, he complains about not sleeping and his speech is slow. She asks John about his mood. He says that he feels life is not worth living, since he cannot work or play sports with his sons like other men. The therapist thinks that John might be experiencing an episode of depression and she writes to his GP, asking that his mental state be assessed.

John starts taking antidepressant medication. After about three weeks, the occupational therapist observes that his mood has begun to improve and that he is more active. She continues to monitor his mood, function and progress for the remaining weeks of pulmonary rehabilitation.

What is assessed

The occupational therapy assessment seeks to elicit information that will enable the therapist to: identify the client's strengths and problem areas; make decisions about intervention; monitor changes in the client's occupational performance, and determine when the intervention should be terminated. This information may be found in any part of the client's life-world, as represented by the European conceptual framework:

- the internal world, which consists of the individual's energy source for action and personal requisites for action

- the external world, which consists of the social contract for action and the place for action

- the interface between the internal and external worlds, where action takes place. This interface consists of the individual's actions, types of action, structuring action and boundaries to action.

The therapist does not look at all these areas with every client but makes clinical decisions about which areas to focus on. The initial assessment and broad functional assessment often indicate where the client's main needs and problems are located so that the therapist can quickly focus on those areas for more detailed assessment. An example of this is given in Example 13.2.

Example 13.2: Moving from functional assessment to detailed assessment

When John is first referred for energy conservation advice, the occupational therapist's initial assessment is designed to build a profile of his daily activities. The therapist asks John if any of these activities cause him particular difficulty, which activities are most important to him and if there are any additional activities he would like to be doing.

John says that getting showered and dressed is a problem because he is often left so tired that he has to rest for an hour or more afterwards. Having identified the occupational performance area that John wants to work on, the therapist then takes him through his hygiene and dressing routine in detail. First, she focuses on the activities of showering and dressing, carrying out a task analysis to identify the components and task sequence. She then discusses the issue of independence with John, in order to find out what level of support would be acceptable to him.

The occupational therapist analyses and interprets the information gained from this assessment in order to work out how John's hygiene and dressing routine might be adapted to use less energy. In this way, she is able to target her first energy conservation advice at the main area of need identified by John himself, thus ensuring maximum impact on his performance and satisfaction.

The European conceptual framework shows us that the therapist does not look only at actions in the interface between the individual's internal and external worlds. It may also be necessary to assess aspects of both the internal and external worlds, as well as the interface, in order to understand the difficulties a person is having with occupational performance and to find solutions that will work for him.

During a course of intervention, the therapist may focus attention on any aspect of the client's performance, assessing those factors that are most relevant at each stage of the process. For example, the client's priority for action may be to achieve independence in personal activities of daily living, so the therapist begins by assessing the factors that are relevant to his performance in this area. Once the client's first goal has been reached, his second goal may be to achieve greater mobility, so the therapist then carries out a more detailed assessment of those aspects of performance that impact on his mobility.

In addition to moving her focus of attention around the conceptual framework, the occupational therapist also shifts from considering broader aspects of the client's occupational performance across a range of performance areas to assessing the precise details of his occupational performance components, and back again, as shown in Figure 13.1.

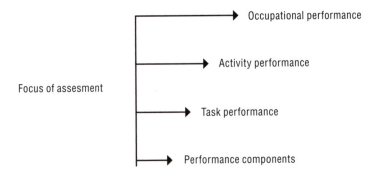

Figure 13.1: Shifting the focus of assessment during an intervention (adapted from Creek 2003)

This shift of perspective, in and out, from large-scale to small-scale and back, 'happens many times during an intervention, often without the therapist's conscious awareness' (Creek 2003, p.18). An example of this is given in Example 13.3.

Example 13.3: Shifting the focus of assessment

Before the occupational therapist gives John advice on energy conservation, she carries out a broad functional assessment to identify the performance area he wants to work on first (assessing occupational performance). When John says that his main problem is with getting showered and dressed in the mornings, the therapist narrows the focus of her assessment so that she can explore the nature of John's difficulties with these activities in more depth (assessing activity performance). By carrying out a task analysis of the activities, the therapist is able to see that John's showering and dressing routine could be simplified by cutting out a number of unnecessary tasks and changing how other tasks are performed, thus conserving his energy (assessing task performance). She then seeks more information about the factors that influence his performance, including performance components and environment, so that she can design a new routine that will work for John (assessing performance components).

After a week, the therapist sees John again to assess how effective the energy conservation advice has been. She first asks if he has been able to make the suggested changes to how he showers and dresses (assessing performance components). She then checks if he is able to manage all the tasks involved in the new daily routine (assessing task performance) and if he is finding that the new routine makes showering and dressing easier (assessing activity performance). Finally, she asks if John now needs less rest after showering and dressing than he did using his original routine, and if he is satisfied with his rate of progress (assessing occupational performance).

Each time the therapist sees John, she shifts her assessment between a broader and narrower focus in order to make sure that proposed changes to performance components and task sequence are having the desired effect on activity and occupational performance.

EVALUATION

As described in the last section, the terms *evaluation* and *assessment* are sometimes used interchangeably, or one is chosen for use rather than the other. However, it is useful to distinguish between them because the concepts they represent are both needed when trying to understand the process of measuring action. While *assessment* is a process of collecting, analysing and interpreting information, *evaluation* means making judgements about the worth of that information.

What the term evaluation means in common usage

In common usage, *evaluation* means 'assessment of worth' (*Shorter Oxford English Dictionary* 2002). For example, critically appraising a research article means making an evaluation of its relevance, quality and value. Evaluation involves making a judgement about something, and that judgement can be about amount, quality or value.

How occupational therapists use the term evaluation

The term evaluation is widely used by occupational therapists to refer to:

the process of using clinical reasoning, problem analysis, self-appraisal and review to interpret the results of assessment in order to make judgements about the situation or needs of an individual, the success of occupational therapy or the therapist's own performance. (Creek 2003, p.53)

From this definition, it can be seen that the occupational therapist might make an evaluation of several aspects of practice:

- the situation or needs of the client – for example, Laver Fawcett (2007, p.6) wrote that evaluation 'involves the collection of data to enable the therapist to make a judgement about…level of independence in an activity of daily living'

- the intervention – for example, Creek (2008, p.68) stated that 'Evaluation is essential to demonstrate the effectiveness of intervention for the client, the therapist, the referring agent and other interested parties'

- the therapist's own performance – for example, Fleming (1994, p.131) described how occupational therapists carry out 'some sort of monitoring and evaluation process…not only observing and analyzing their patients' behavior, but their own as well'

- the service – for example, Corr (2003, p.235) pointed out that 'unless occupational therapists evaluate their services, they will not know if the service is meeting its aims and objectives'.

The process of evaluating the degree of change following an intervention is called outcome measurement. Outcome measurement is 'evaluation of the nature and degree of change brought about by intervention, or the extent to which a goal has been reached or an outcome has been achieved' (Creek 2003, p.56).

Creek (2008) described evaluation as part of the process of reviewing interventions and services to ensure that they are fit for purpose and to safeguard standards. She argued that 'evaluation of services should be carried out by occupational therapists themselves against their own standards of performance' (p.68). According to Finlay (1997, p.178), evaluation should be a central component of practice because 'our integrity and confidence as therapists is derived from our ability to evaluate what we do'. Duncan (2006, p.55) went further in describing the evaluation of occupational therapy as 'an ethical and professional imperative'.

The European understanding of the term evaluation

· ·

Evaluation is the process of obtaining, interpreting and appraising information in order to prioritize problems and needs, to plan and modify interventions and to judge the worth of interventions.

· ·

This definition was constructed from seven elements taken from definitions of *evaluation* found in the occupational therapy literature:

- a process

- obtaining information

- interpreting information

- appraising information

- in order to prioritize problems and needs

- in order to plan and modify interventions

- in order to judge the worth of interventions.

As described above, a process is 'a continuous series of actions, events or changes' (*Shorter Oxford English Dictionary* 2002). The actions that make up the process of evaluation are obtaining, interpreting and appraising information. The process of evaluation is circular rather than linear, as interpretation of information may lead to the need to obtain more information. This circular process is shown in Example 13.4.

To obtain is to 'secure or gain as the result of request or effort' (*Shorter Oxford English Dictionary* 2002). To appraise is to 'estimate the amount, quality, or excellence' of something (*ibid.*). To interpret is to explain to oneself or to obtain significant information from something (*ibid.*). The occupational therapist gains information through the processes of data gathering and assessment and then, having estimated that the information is of a high enough quality, she decides on the significance of the information to the situation under consideration. This process is illustrated in Example 13.4.

Example 13.4: Evaluation of the effectiveness of intervention

The first pulmonary rehabilitation programme that John attends includes weekly sessions of individualized advice on energy conservation from the occupational therapist. At the beginning of each session, the occupational therapist obtains information from John that will enable her to evaluate the effectiveness of the previous week's session. This includes information about: the relevance of the advice to his particular circumstances; the degree to which he has been able to apply the advice and make changes to his daily patterns of activity; how much improvement he has experienced in his task, activity and occupational performance, and the extent to which he feels that his personal goals have been met.

While obtaining this information, the therapist appraises it for its relevance and reliability. Suspecting that John might be overstating his degree of improvement, she asks his wife how she sees the change in John's performance. The therapist then interprets the significance of what John and his wife have told her and makes a judgement about John's level of improvement. This becomes the starting point for planning what further information to give John.

When the therapist evaluates assessment information, she does so in order to be able to:

- decide which of the client's problems and needs should be addressed first

- plan interventions to solve those problems or meet identified needs, and modify interventions in the light of ongoing assessment results

- judge the worth of interventions by their effectiveness and cost-effectiveness.

These functions of the occupational therapist's evaluation of client data are illustrated in the case described in Examples 13.1 to 13.4.

SUMMARY

This chapter has explored the skills that the occupational therapist uses in order to: reach an understanding of the occupational performance of individuals, groups and communities; identify strengths and weaknesses in that performance, and plan and monitor interventions. These skills are *assessment* and *evaluation*.

Evaluation, as defined in this chapter, is 'a component of a broader assessment process' (Laver Fawcett 2007, p.6). Assessment is a process of collecting, analysing and interpreting information. Evaluation involves not only obtaining information but also interpreting and appraising it, that is, making judgements about amount (such as the degree of change following intervention) and/or value (such as the cost-effectiveness of an intervention).

Chapter 12 described the skills of task analysis, activity analysis and occupational mapping which, together, enable the occupational therapist to reach a deep understanding of occupations and activities. This chapter explained how the skills of assessment and evaluation enable the therapist to understand occupational performance. Chapter 14 illustrates how all these skills are implemented in designing therapeutic interventions for occupational therapy clients.

REFERENCES

Corr, S. (2003) 'Evaluate, evaluate, evaluate.' *British Journal of Occupational Therapy 66*, 6, 235.

Creek, J. (2003) *Occupational Therapy Defined as a Complex Intervention.* London: College of Occupational Therapists.

Creek, J. (2008) 'Approaches to practice.' In J. Creek and L. Lougher (eds) *Occupational Therapy and Mental Health, Fourth Edition.* Edinburgh: Churchill Livingstone Elsevier.

Creek, J. and Bullock, A. (2008) 'Assessment and outcome measurement.' In J. Creek and L. Lougher (eds) *Occupational Therapy and Mental Health, Fourth Edition.* Edinburgh: Churchill Livingstone Elsevier.

Creek, J. and Lougher, L. (2008) *Occupational Therapy and Mental Health, Fourth Edition.* Edinburgh: Churchill Livingstone Elsevier.

Duncan, E.A.S. (2006) 'Skills and processes in occupational therapy.' In E.A.S. Duncan (ed.) *Foundations for Practice in Occupational Therapy.* Edinburgh: Elsevier Churchill Livingstone.

Finlay, L. (1997) *The Practice of Psychosocial Occupational Therapy, Second Edition.* Cheltenham: Stanley Thornes.

Fleming, M.H. (1994) 'The therapist with the three-track mind.' In C. Mattingly and M.H. Fleming (eds.) *Clinical Reasoning: Forms of Inquiry in a Therapeutic Practice.* Philadelphia, PA: F.A. Davis.

Hagedorn, R. (2001) *Foundations for Practice in Occupational Therapy, Third Edition.* Edinburgh: Churchill Livingstone.

Laver Fawcett, A.J. (2007) *Principles of Assessment and Outcome Measurement for Occupational Therapists and Physiotherapists: Theory, Skills and Application.* Chichester: Wiley.

Macdonald, E.M. (1976) *Occupational Therapy in Rehabilitation, Fourth Edition.* London: Ballière Tindall.

Mattingly, C. (1994) 'Occupational therapy as a two-body practice: the lived body.' In C. Mattingly and M.H. Fleming *Clinical Reasoning: Forms of Inquiry in a Therapeutic Practice.* Philadelphia, PA: F.D. Davis.

Mosey, A.C. (1986) *Psychosocial Components of Occupational Therapy.* New York: Raven Press.

Neistadt, M.E. (1998) 'Introduction to evaluation and interviewing.' In M.E. Neistadt and E.B. Crepeau (eds) *Willard and Spackman's Occupational Therapy, Ninth Edition.* Philadelphia, PA: Lippincott.

Shorter Oxford English Dictionary, Fifth Edition (2002) Oxford: Clarendon Press.

Sumsion, T. (1999) 'The client-centred approach.' In T. Sumsion (ed.) *Client-centred Practice in Occupational Therapy: A Guide to Implementation.* Edinburgh: Churchill Livingstone.

CHAPTER 14

FACILITATING ACTION

INTRODUCTION

The European conceptual framework for occupational therapy defines 25 key occupational therapy concepts and explains how they relate to each other, as shown in Figure 14.1. The framework is intended to provide a conceptual foundation for theory building, as discussed in Chapter 3, and for occupational therapy practice.

Chapter 12 described how the conceptual framework underpins the core occupational therapy skills of *task analysis, activity analysis* and *occupational mapping*. Chapter 13 discussed how the conceptual framework can inform *assessment* and *evaluation*. This chapter will explain how the conceptual framework can guide the occupational therapist's thinking throughout the intervention process.

The title of the chapter is 'Facilitating Action'. To facilitate means to 'make easy or easier; promote, help forward' (*Shorter Oxford English Dictionary* 2002). By their interventions, occupational therapists aim to promote or help forward their clients' occupations by making task and activity performance easier.

The chapter begins with the story of Felicity, which is outlined in Example 14.1. This story will be used throughout the chapter to illustrate occupational therapy intervention based on the European conceptual framework. The chapter takes the reader through the process of intervention, from referral to discharge, highlighting how the therapist's reasoning and decision making are guided by the conceptual framework.

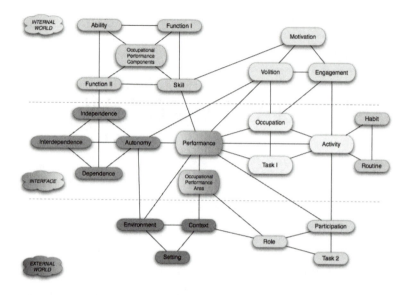

Figure 14.1: The European conceptual framework for occupational therapy

Example 14.1: Felicity's story

Felicity is a 45-year-old white British woman, living in her own house in a town in the north of England. She has an older, married sister who lives about 80 miles away. Their parents died eight years ago, within a few months of each other.

Felicity left school at age 18 with three 'A'-levels and went to university to study sociology. In her second year, she became depressed and took an overdose of aspirin. She recovered and finished her course to gain a second class degree. She then spent a year travelling in China and the Far East. Upon returning home, she took a series of casual jobs, working as a dental receptionist, a chambermaid in a hotel and an assistant in a day centre for children with learning disabilities. Eventually, she decided to go back to university to become a nurse for people with learning disabilities. During the course, Felicity had another episode of depression. Her GP prescribed antidepressant medication and she was able to complete her studies.

After the death of her parents, Felicity had her first psychotic episode. She became severely depressed and thought that she had killed her father by something she said. Her GP referred her to a psychiatrist who diagnosed bipolar disorder. He prescribed antidepressant medication and said that Felicity should continue to take it for the rest of her life.

Felicity describes herself as heterosexual and has had several boyfriends. However, she has never married, or lived with a man, and she has never been pregnant. She has a wide circle of friends and enjoys a range of activities, including reading, going to the theatre, walking and knitting. Felicity belongs to a book club and has recently joined a knitting group, which meets once a week. She loves travelling and describes herself as 'restless'. Between jobs, she usually goes travelling for a few weeks.

Unlike her sister, who has always lived in the same town, Felicity moves to a different area every few years, often following an episode of depression and usually to take up a new job. She bought her present house five years ago but has changed jobs while living there. She is currently working full time as a lecturer at the local university.

The university was reorganized recently and the nursing programme moved from the School of Medicine to the School of Health Sciences. The new Dean wants to raise the research profile of the school and is encouraging staff to bid for research funding. Staff who do not have PhDs are expected to take on more teaching to give their colleagues time for research activity.

Since Felicity does not have a research degree, she has been given a heavier teaching load, including two new subjects. She feels stressed and believes that the Dean is trying to pressure her to leave because she does not have a PhD. She finds it hard to concentrate and wakes early in the morning, worrying about her workload. Her appetite has diminished and she makes excuses not to see her friends. She thinks that people are talking about her, saying that she smells and should not be allowed into the university.

The leader of the nursing programme, who has known Felicity for a long time, recognizes that she is becoming ill and suggests that she should see her GP. The GP signs her off work and refers her to a psychiatrist at the local hospital.

OCCUPATIONAL THERAPY INTERVENTION

Occupational therapy is concerned with 'the nature, balance, pattern and context of occupations in individual lives' (Creek 2003, p.31). The overall goal of intervention is 'for the client to achieve a satisfying performance and balance of occupations…that will support recovery, health, well being and social participation' (p.32).

Occupational therapy intervention consists of a number of stages that are carried out by the therapist in collaboration with the client and relevant others. Intervention is sometimes described as a linear or circular process, in which each stage is succeeded by the next one in a logical sequence, as shown in Figure 14.2. In practice, these stages may be carried out in almost any order, may be carried out simultaneously and may be repeated as often as necessary.

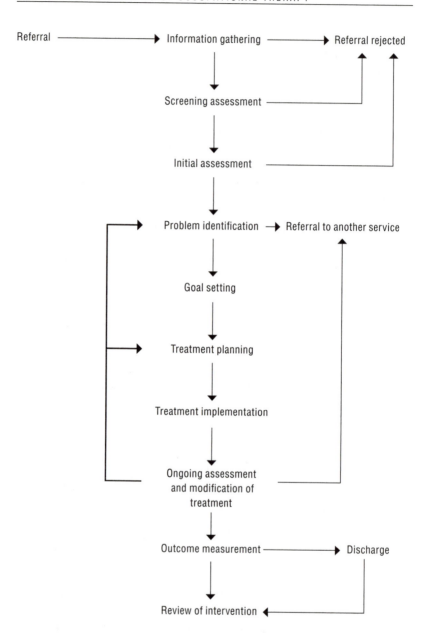

Figure 14.2: The occupational therapy process

Initial assessment and problem identification

Occupational therapy intervention begins when the client is referred to the occupational therapist, or when the therapist first meets the client. At this point in the process, the therapist begins to gather information about the client in order to understand his problems or needs. Information collected at this stage may be from any of the clusters in the conceptual framework, although the therapist is more likely to look at the client's occupations and occupational performance before focusing in on performance components and environments.

When the therapist and client meet, the therapist begins to add information to that which has already been obtained, and starts to map the client's occupations. An example of information gathering and the initial interview is given in Example 14.2, which describes what happens when a community occupational therapist is asked to see Felicity.

Example 14.2: Gathering information about Felicity

Felicity is discussed at the weekly referral meeting of the community mental health team (CMHT) and the psychiatrist says that he will review her medication. Team members agree that the occupational therapist, Michelle, is the most appropriate person to coordinate Felicity's care because her immediate problems are practical ones to do with her work and activities of daily life. The therapist arranges to see Felicity when she comes for her appointment with the psychiatrist.

Prior to this meeting, the therapist reads the GP referral letter and Felicity's case notes. She discovers that Felicity has had contact with mental health services in the past, that she is single and that she is a learning disabilities nurse. Michelle forms the impression that Felicity functions well when her mood is normal but her occupational performance deteriorates across all areas when she is depressed.

At their first meeting, the therapist hopes to elicit Felicity's feelings about accepting mental health services, so she explores aspects of the energy source for action and social contract for action clusters: *motivation, volition, role* and *task 2.* She finds out that Felicity's motivation to engage in treatment is not strong, due to her feelings of hopelessness, her fatigue and her poor concentration. However, she is willing to accept the patient role because her sister is very anxious about her and has made it clear that she expects Felicity to comply with whatever treatment is offered.

Michelle also wants to find out more about Felicity's usual range of occupations, the ones she is currently having difficulty with and whether she is getting any support. The focus of her questions is on the action and boundaries to action clusters: *performance, occupational performance areas* and *dependence.* Michelle asks Felicity about the range of activities she performs on a normal day, confirming her impression that Felicity engages in an appropriate range of occupations when she is well but is having problems in all occupational performance areas at the moment.

At some point in the initial assessment, the therapist and client reach a decision about whether or not they want to work together. If either of them feels that occupational therapy intervention is inappropriate at this time, the therapist will inform the referring agent that the referral is not accepted, giving the reasons (Creek 2003). If the therapist and client decide to proceed with the intervention, the therapist continues to gather information about the client. She also works with the client to identify which problems they are going to work on, and formulates these problems into outcome goals. Example 14.3 describes how the occupational therapist works with Felicity to identify which problems she wants to address first.

The purpose of the initial assessment is not only to enable the therapist to formulate the client's problems but also, and equally importantly, to help the client to understand his own performance and performance deficits. The terms in the European conceptual framework can be used to map the individual's usual, expected or desired occupations so that he can identify for himself where the problems are and what he hopes to gain from occupational therapy.

Example 14.3: Identifying Felicity's problems

In order to find out more about the difficulties that Felicity is having at present, Michelle focuses her attention on the forms of action, personal requisites for action and place for action clusters: *occupation, activity, task 1, performance components, function 2* and *social environment*. This assessment begins at the initial interview and continues during subsequent meetings, most of which take place at Felicity's house.

Felicity is sleeping badly; she feels physically and mentally exhausted; she finds it hard to shop, cook or eat; her personal hygiene is poor, and she avoids seeing her friends, if possible. She spends her time either lying in bed, ruminating about how terrible she feels, or wandering around the house, unable to settle to any particular activity. Her sister visits at least once a week, bringing fresh food. She encourages Felicity to wash and change her clothes, cleans the house and cooks a meal, which she insists that Felicity eats with her.

Felicity's problems can be seen in the action interface: her normal habits and routines have broken down and she is unable to perform her usual range of occupations. However, Michelle reasons that the cause of these problems is located in Felicity's internal world: depression is interfering with both her energy source for action and personal requisites for action: *motivation, volition, engagement* and *function 2*.

Goal setting and treatment planning

As the therapist identifies what she thinks are the client's problems, she checks with him to find out if his perceptions match hers or if he disagrees. Setting goals for intervention can be straightforward but it can also be a protracted process of negotiation and compromise, especially if the client has multiple and complex needs.

The long-term goals of occupational therapy intervention are to improve occupational performance. It may not be possible to set long-term goals at the start of the intervention, either because the client is not able to make an autonomous decision or because the therapist does not have enough information. In either case, the therapist sets short-term, time-limited goals and reviews them on an agreed date. Short-term goals may be to develop occupational performance components, or may be in any other area of the conceptual framework. When they have been achieved, the therapist sets new short-term goals or, if possible, agrees long-term goals with the client.

If the client needs to make a lot of changes in order to meet his long-term goals, the therapist may decide to set intermediate goals so that progress towards long-term goals can be measured. For example, the client's long-term goal may be improvement in an area of occupational performance but the intermediate goals are to develop performance components to support that performance.

As described in Chapter 13, the therapist's focus of attention moves between different clusters of the conceptual framework as new information is obtained or in response to changes in the client's performance. The therapist's attention also shifts between a wider perspective of the client's occupational performance and a narrower focus on activity performance, task performance and performance components, as she identifies the precise problem area or evaluates the effects of interventions.

Effective occupational therapy intervention is highly individualized, therefore a unique treatment plan is devised for each client. The therapist uses her skills of task analysis and activity analysis to select activities that are within the client's capabilities and that will enable him to develop the desired performance components and performance. The therapist also considers the client's motivation and volition so that she can identify activities to maintain his engagement throughout the therapeutic process. It may also be necessary for the therapist to analyse the client's physical and social environments to determine if any modifications are needed.

The treatment plan includes the goals of intervention, the proposed timescale for reassessment, the proposed treatment and the person or persons responsible for carrying it out.

The process of negotiating the first set of goals with Felicity and planning interventions to meet those goals is described in Example 14.4.

Example 14.4: Setting goals and planning intervention with Felicity

At this stage in her depressive cycle, Felicity is not able to identify any personal goals, other than wanting to get better. Michelle suggests that Felicity will feel better if she is able to establish a more normal daily routine, incorporating sleep, personal care, eating properly, seeing other people and, if possible, engaging in activities that she enjoys. Felicity agrees and, after some discussion, they decide to start working on her sleep, personal hygiene and eating, which Felicity feels are the areas causing most distress. The goal is to re-establish a normal daily routine of sleeping, personal care and eating.

Michelle wants to identify exactly what difficulties Felicity is having with these three occupations so that she can plan effective interventions. Her assessment now focuses on aspects of the structuring action, personal requisites for action and energy source for action clusters. Felicity has the abilities and skills necessary for carrying out her daily activities; the problem is that she lacks the energy to perform (*motivation*) and the structure of her life has been disrupted (*routine*), so that she has difficulty translating performance components into effective action (*function 2*).

Most of the conversations between Felicity and the occupational therapist take place in her house. The therapist visits three times a week and on each visit they agree on an activity to perform together, such as doing the washing up or making a simple meal. Michelle elicits the information she wants by asking questions and getting Felicity to perform specific tasks. By observing Felicity's current performance, Michelle is able to set a baseline from which to measure changes during the intervention.

Michelle and Felicity together explore what is blocking Felicity's ability to carry out her normal daily routines. As part of this process, Michelle carries out a task analysis of Felicity's normal bedtime routine and Felicity is able to identify which parts of that routine have broken down. They then discuss alternative approaches to re-establishing Felicity's routines so that she can choose the one she thinks will work best for her.

Michelle is aware that Felicity experiences recurrent episodes of severe depression so she wants to provide Felicity with ways of coping that she can use on future occasions, not just during this episode.

Treatment implementation

When the goals of intervention have been agreed, and a treatment plan drawn up, the plan is implemented. In reality, it is likely that treatment will have begun when the therapist and client first meet. The client-centred practice of occupational therapy involves the client from the start in identifying needs, setting priorities and choosing treatment media, 'thus increasing the client's responsibility, choice, autonomy and control over her/his care' (Creek 2003, p.8).

The main legitimate tools of occupational therapy practice are activity and environmental modification (Creek 2003). The client's performance of activities during therapy is intended to: develop performance components; build motivation and volition; establish or re-establish healthy habits and routines; promote appropriate interdependence; change environments, and enable participation in society. Modifications to the physical and social environments, which may be temporary or permanent, are intended to enable and support the occupational performance of the client.

Intervention may focus on any area of the client's internal world, external world or action interface, but is likely to include elements of all three. The therapist is concerned with the client's occupational performance (interface) but, in order to achieve effective performance, she may: help him to develop new skills (internal world); modify his physical environment (external world); help him to develop more efficient habits (interface); recommend a higher level of support (external world), and so on.

The process of treatment implementation with Felicity is described in Example 14.5.

Example 14.5: Implementing treatment with Felicity

Felicity's main motivation for engaging in occupational therapy is that she wants to relieve her sister's anxiety. The occupational therapist knows that this will change as the new medication takes effect and Felicity's depression starts to lift. For now, she accepts that Felicity has low energy levels and does not experience pleasure in what she does. Michelle has to provide the energy for action at this stage of treatment by giving clear directions and working alongside Felicity. As Felicity's mood improves and her fatigue lifts, she will find it easier to carry out her daily activities.

Treatment includes aspects of Felicity's internal and external worlds, as well as the action interface. In the internal world, the therapist wants to improve Felicity's: energy for engaging in activity (*motivation*); ability to initiate and maintain action (*volition*), and interest in what she is doing (*engagement*). In the external world, Michelle wants to help Felicity to: perform her daily activities at the appropriate time (*temporal environment*); clean and tidy up while performing activities such as cooking (*physical environment* and *setting*); utilize whatever social support is available (*sociocultural environment* and *role*), and do her own shopping (*participation* and *role*). In the action interface, Michelle wants to help Felicity to: perform the activities of sleeping, washing and eating every day (*performance* and *routine*); accept that she temporarily needs help to manage her personal care and household tasks (*dependence*), and eventually enable her to perform her daily activities without assistance (*independence*).

While working with Felicity on re-establishing a healthy pattern of daily activities, the therapist gives her tools that she will be able to use during future episodes of depression. For example, Michelle suggests that Felicity should think about which activities are most important for maintaining health and well-being during a depressive episode and use her limited energy to perform those activities rather than others. She advises Felicity to keep a CD player by the bed and listen to a story to stop herself ruminating if she has a bout of insomnia. This removes some of the anxiety from not being able to sleep. Michelle also helps Felicity to identify potential sources of help and support, and advises her to put support in place before she becomes too depressed, if she feels another episode coming on.

Ongoing assessment and treatment modification

Throughout treatment implementation, the therapist monitors the client's performance through observation and assessment. Attention may be paid to any aspect of the action interface, the internal world or the external world. This continual monitoring and evaluation of the effects of intervention allows the therapist to make ongoing modifications to the intervention, the treatment plan or the goals, in response to the client's immediate needs.

As described above, the therapist also changes her focus, from the client's occupational performance to his performance components and back again, during the course of an intervention. This shift of focus allows her to see whether improvements in performance components are translated into improvements in task, activity and occupational performance. If the client is developing new skills but is not using them to perform satisfactorily, then the therapist looks at other areas of the conceptual framework to see what is interfering with performance. For example, there may be environmental or social barriers blocking the individual's occupational performance. In order to increase the client's autonomy, the therapist helps him to identify barriers and work out ways of dealing with them.

The process of ongoing assessment and treatment modification with Felicity is described in Example 14.6.

Example 14.6: Ongoing assessment during Felicity's treatment programme

When Michelle and Felicity agreed the goals of intervention, Michelle suggested that they should review progress in four weeks' time. She expected that the new medication would be taking effect by then and that Felicity would be starting to sleep better.

As described in Example 14.4, the occupational therapist visits Felicity at home three times a week and is able to watch her performing some of her usual daily life activities. By closely observing Felicity, Michelle is able to judge how much support to give and when her input can be reduced. Michelle pays attention not only to Felicity's activity performance and routines but also to other areas of the conceptual framework: her energy levels (*motivation*); her level of interest in what she is doing (*engagement*); how much prompting she needs to begin and complete activities (*volition*); how much help she needs (*dependence*), and how effectively she performs activities (*function 2*).

When the first set of goals is reviewed after four weeks, Felicity has made progress with sleeping, personal hygiene and eating, although she is not performing these occupations to her normal standard. Together, Michelle and Felicity set new goals to increase Felicity's range of activities and agree to review progress again in four weeks. Michelle reduces the number of weekly sessions to two, anticipating that Felicity will be able to maintain her current level of performance with less support.

The second review indicates that Felicity is continuing to make progress in all areas of occupational performance. Her mood has improved (*performance component*) and she has more energy (*motivation*). She feels more able to make decisions (*volition*) and is less dependent on her sister and Michelle to buy food and advise her what to cook (*independence*).

Michelle and Felicity have a review meeting with the psychiatrist and agree that Felicity will aim to return to work in another four weeks. She contacts her head of department and arranges for a graded return to work, starting two days a week and gradually increasing to full time.

Final assessment and outcome measurement

At the time when the occupational therapist and the client negotiate the goals of intervention, they agree on a date when those goals will be reviewed. The length of an intervention before the goals are reviewed depends on how much change the client needs to make to reach them. In some cases, a goal may be reached within a single session; in other cases, it may take weeks or months to achieve a goal.

At the review interview, the therapist repeats the original assessment with the client and compares the present score with the baseline assessment. The difference between the baseline score and the present score indicates the amount of change that has taken place during the course of intervention.

As described above, goals may be set in any area of the conceptual framework, so change can be measured in any area. However, the overall goal of occupational therapy intervention is to improve occupational performance. The therapist and client evaluate the client's progress against the goals of the intervention to determine if those goals have been fully met, partially met or not met at all. This is the outcome of the intervention.

The final assessment and outcomes of intervention with Felicity are described in Example 14.7.

Example 14.7: Final assessment and outcomes of intervention with Felicity

During the last four weeks of the intervention, the therapist sees Felicity once a week, at the CMHT offices. Their last meeting takes place the week before Felicity is due to return to work. Her facial expression is brighter and she is well groomed. She says that she is anxious about returning to work but her head of department is being supportive and her colleagues have sent her flowers.

Michelle reminds Felicity about the original goals of occupational therapy intervention and asks if she has any remaining difficulties. Felicity says that she is sleeping reasonably well and that she has put on some of the weight she lost. Her sister no longer comes to see her every week but Felicity has been to stay for a weekend with her sister and brother-in-law. She has also been out with friends on a couple of occasions.

Michelle and Felicity agree that the occupational therapy goals have been met and it is appropriate to end the intervention. Felicity says that she has written down some of the strategies that worked for her and she will try to use them if she gets depressed again.

SUMMARY

The project to define key professional terms for European occupational therapists, begun in 2001, was intended to facilitate communication across the many cultural and linguistic borders that exist within this diverse continent. However, the terminology project eventually led to the development of a distinctively European theory of occupational therapy: the European conceptual framework for occupational therapy.

The worth of a theory can be measured by its ability to produce good results, and the utility of an occupational therapy theory lies in its ease of application, its relevance to practice and, ultimately, the extent to which practitioners find that it improves their work. This chapter has illustrated how the European conceptual framework can be used as a guide to the therapist's reasoning at each stage of the process of intervention. The framework provides a way of managing the complexity of occupational therapy intervention by acknowledging the dynamic nature of people's occupations and avoiding 'the hobgoblin of oversimplification' (Yerxa 1988, p.5) that has dogged the profession for many years.

The reader is recommended to test the utility of the European conceptual framework for her or himself. Find out if the definitions enhance your understanding of occupation and occupational performance. Apply the concepts to your clients' performance and see if they help you, and the client, to make sense of his experiences. Use the terms with your colleagues and judge whether they make communication easier.

Members of the European Network of Occupational Therapy in Higher Education (ENOTHE) terminology project group hope that the European conceptual framework will become a living, growing, developing foundation for occupational therapy theory and practice. It belongs to you.

REFERENCES

Creek, J. (2003) *Occupational Therapy Defined as a Complex Intervention*. London: College of Occupational Therapists.

Shorter Oxford English Dictionary, Fifth Edition (2002) Oxford: Clarendon Press.

Yerxa, E. (1988) 'Oversimplification: the hobgoblin of theory and practice in occupational therapy.' *Canadian Journal of Occupational Therapy 55*, 1, 5–6.

SUBJECT INDEX

AUTHOR INDEX